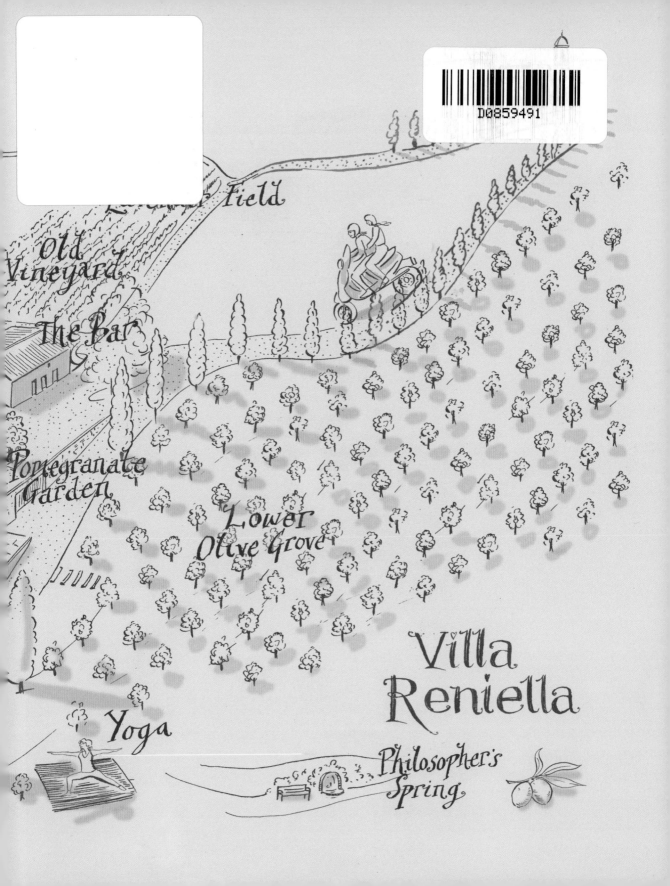

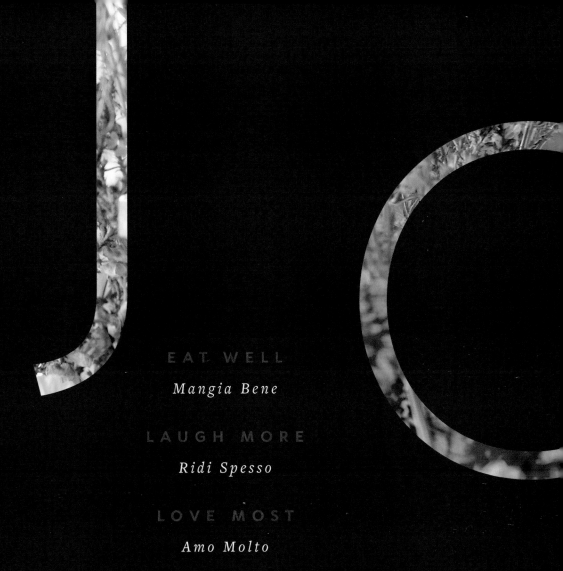

JOY

EAT WELL
Mangia Bene

LAUGH MORE
Ridi Spesso

LOVE MOST
Amo Molto

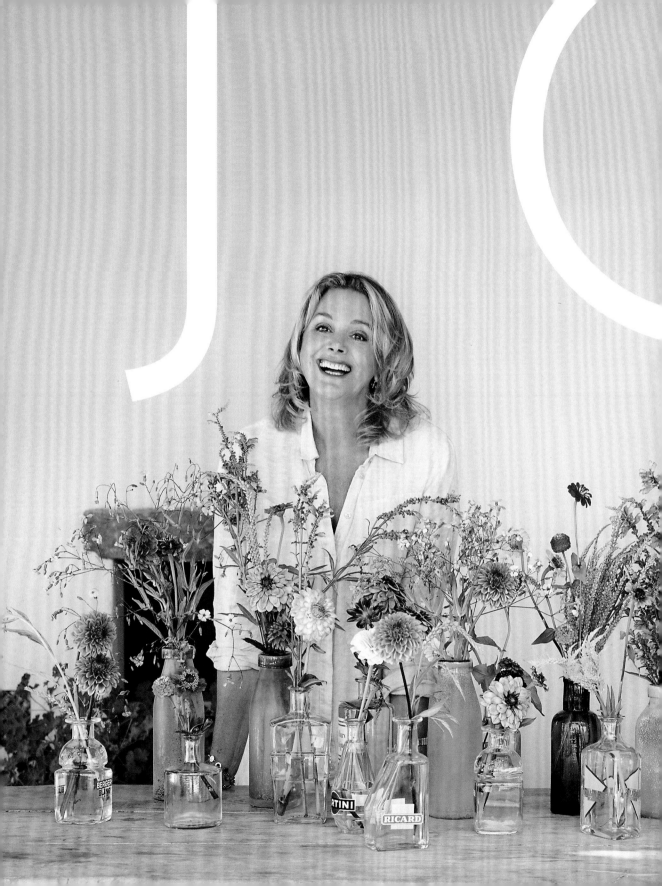

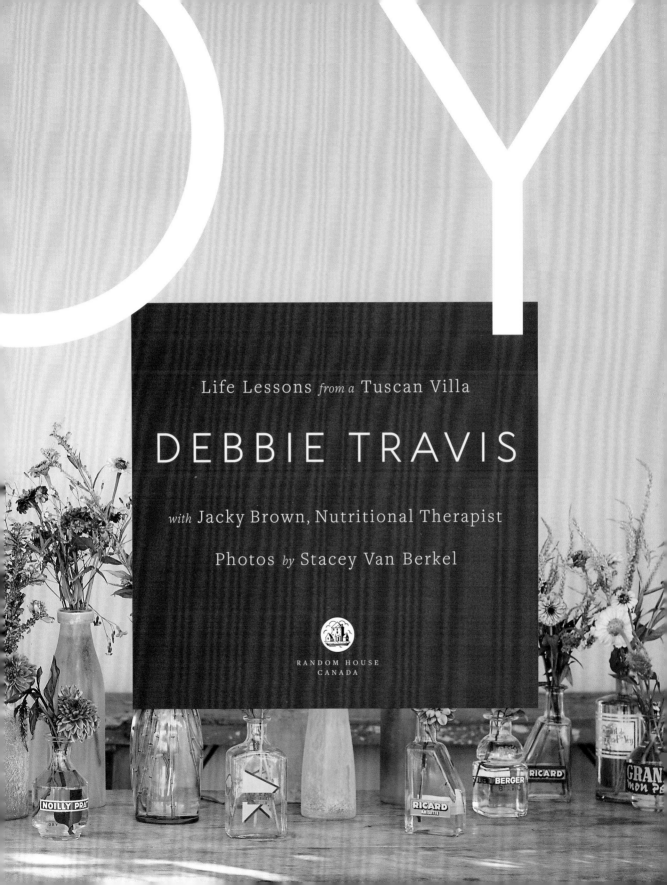

Life Lessons *from a* Tuscan Villa

DEBBIE TRAVIS

with Jacky Brown, Nutritional Therapist

Photos *by* Stacey Van Berkel

RANDOM HOUSE
CANADA

www.penguinrandomhouse.ca

Random House Canada and colophon are registered trademarks.

Library and Archives Canada Cataloguing in Publication

Title: Joy : life lessons from a Tuscan villa / Debbie Travis.
Other titles: Life lessons from a Tuscan villa
Names: Travis, Debbie, author.
Identifiers: Canadiana (print) 20200394614 | Canadiana (ebook) 20200397273 |
    ISBN 9780735280106 (hardcover) | ISBN 9780735280113 (EPUB)
Subjects: LCSH: Joy. | LCSH: Happiness. | LCSH: Health—Popular works.
Classification: LCC BF575.H27 T73 2021 | DDC 158—dc23

ISBN 9780735280106
eBook ISBN 9780735280113

Cover and text design: Lisa Jager
Image credits: Luke Brown, 21, 163; Daniela Cesarie, 20, 93, 94, 97, 98, 117, 136, 149; Max Rosenstein, 33, 36, 142, 144, 156; George Ross, 10, 99. Endpaper map of Villa Reniella by Michael Hill

Printed in China
10 9 8 7 6 5 4 3 2 1

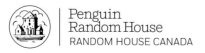

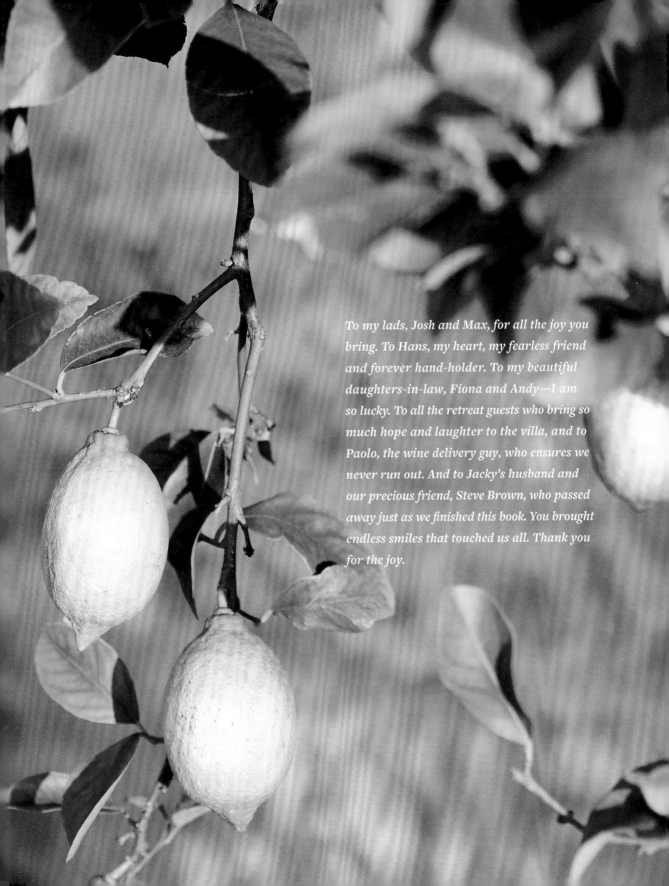

To my lads, Josh and Max, for all the joy you bring. To Hans, my heart, my fearless friend and forever hand-holder. To my beautiful daughters-in-law, Fiona and Andy—I am so lucky. To all the retreat guests who bring so much hope and laughter to the villa, and to Paolo, the wine delivery guy, who ensures we never run out. And to Jacky's husband and our precious friend, Steve Brown, who passed away just as we finished this book. You brought endless smiles that touched us all. Thank you for the joy.

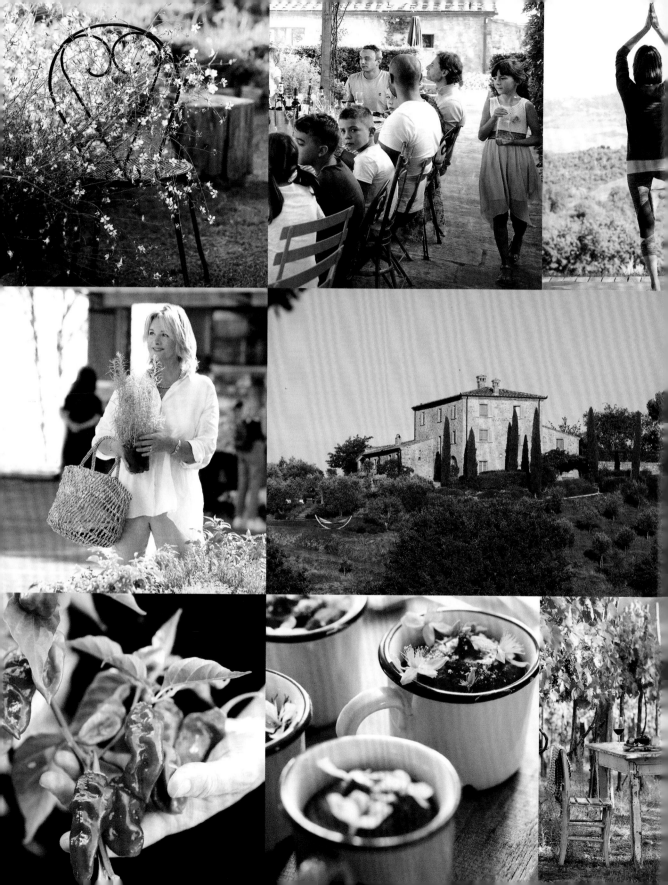

CONTENTS

Ciao Ciao

IF YOU HAPPEN TO BE LOOKING for me this morning, please walk past the kitchen door that is usually ajar, past the geraniums tumbling from mismatched terracotta pots, and head down the stone steps towards the pool. Take a right along the terrace of lemon trees, and feel free to grab a few—they are ready for picking. Chances are you'll meet Eva picking flowers from the enormous oleander bushes and possibly hear the drone of Luca's tractor in the nearby field. Continue following the narrow grass path, but be careful—it is steep in parts. You will soon spot the wooden yoga platform perched over the valley. Stop for a moment to drink in the sweeping views over velvety hills of gilded wheat, dotted with vineyards, rows of grapevines as neat as soldiers lined up and ready for battle. In the distance is the medieval town of Montepulciano, a fortress of butter-coloured stone shimmering in the summer heat. Now take a sharp right past the young olive grove, and there, shaded by a walnut tree, is a rustic wooden hut. The door will be open to let in the scented air, and this is where you'll find me, plonked on a worn leather chair.

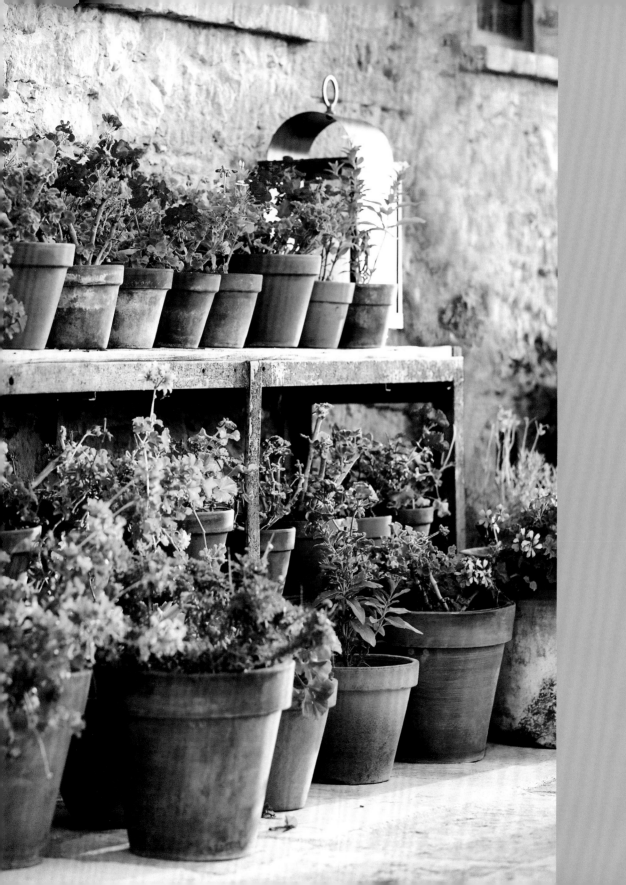

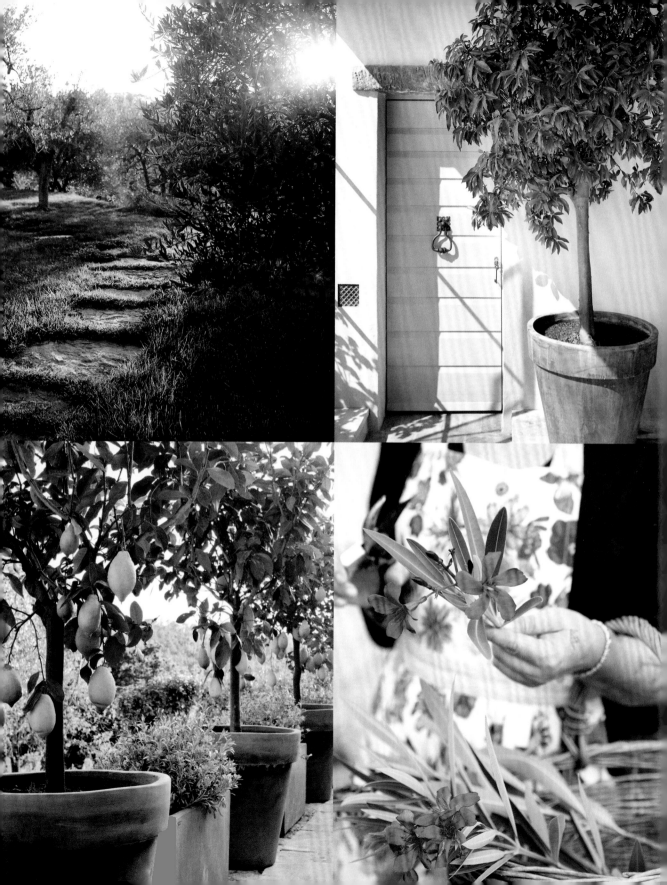

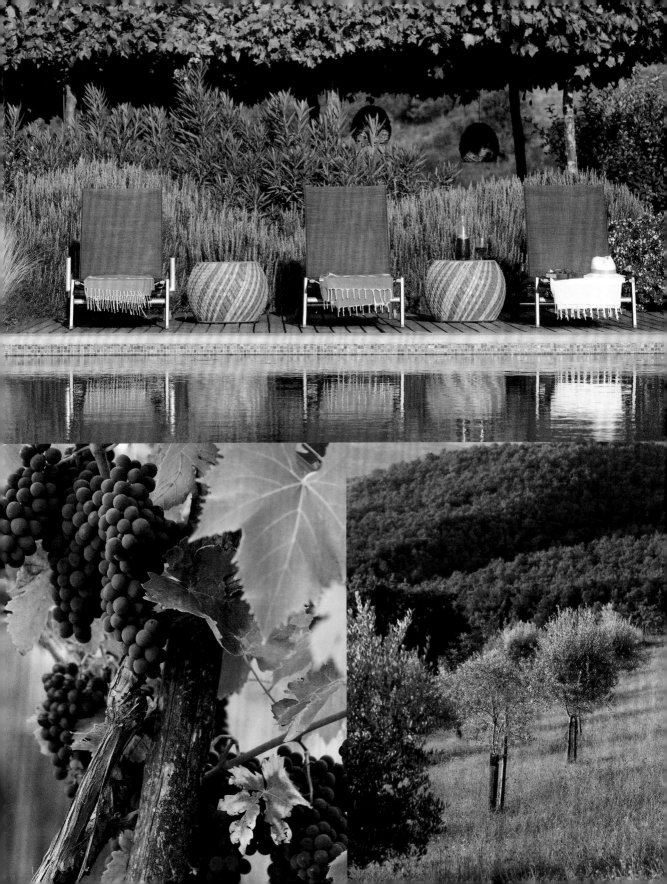

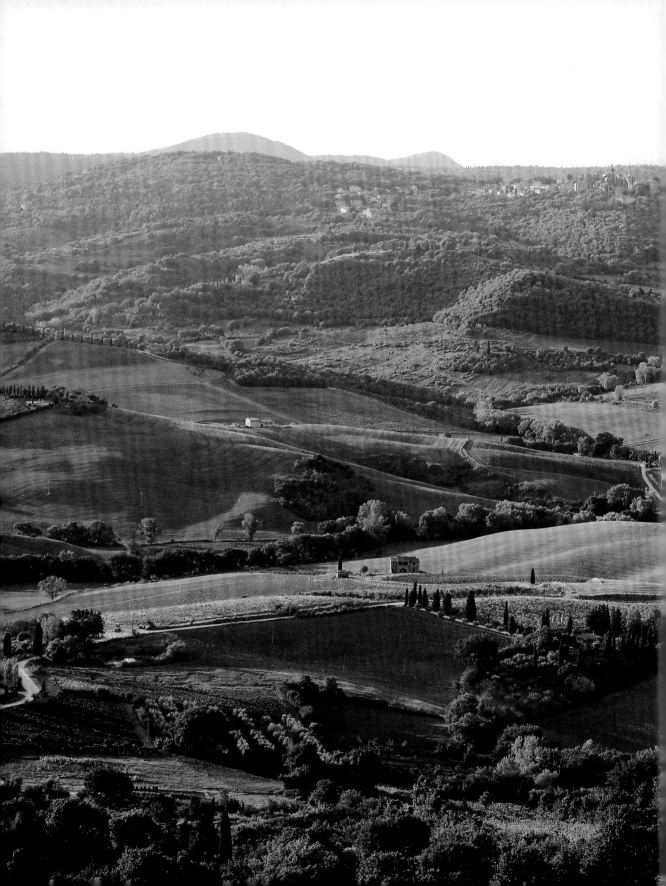

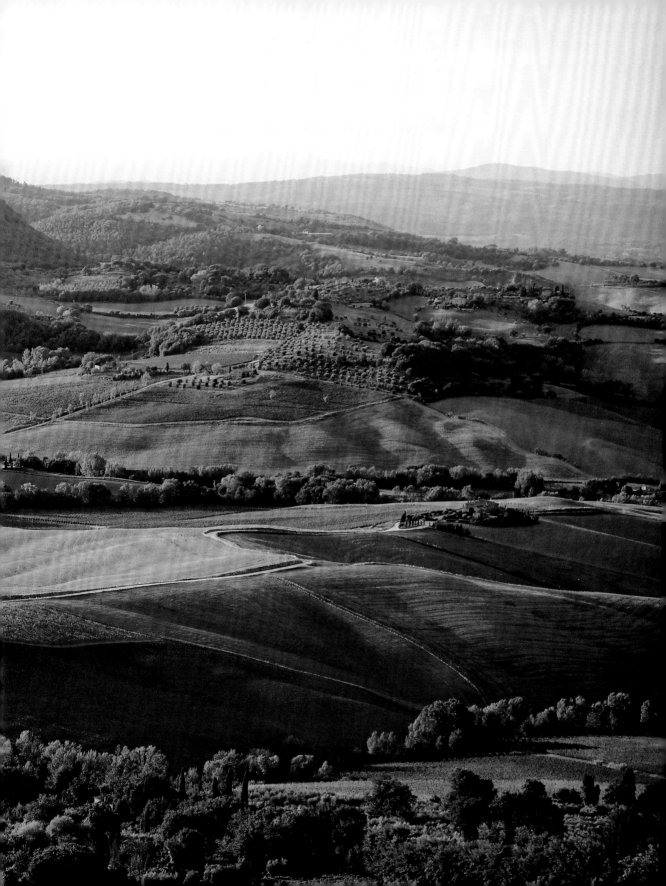

There are three massage huts, built from uneven planks faded to a smoky grey, scattered along the periphery of the gardens of Villa Reniella. On any given day, guests at the retreats I hold here will be kneaded into peaceful oblivion by Lalla, the doors flung open, allowing the breeze to whisper over naked bodies dozing to the sound of summer crickets. I have commandeered the roomiest of the three cabins, replacing the massage table with a desk and stocking the shelves with pens, paper, books and sticky notes. So here I am at my laptop on day one of my new adventure: writing this book. The simple wooden hut is the epitome of peace, just me and my thoughts.

But you have to laugh—this is Italy, after all. Minutes into my solitude, the silence is broken. Fabio, Stefano and Fulvio, some of the remaining *ragazzi* who originally restored the property, have appeared out of nowhere to dig a trench right behind my hut. Initially I'm irritated by the disturbance, but before too long the familiar music of life here swells the heart. The three men laugh along to each other's stories. There is much humming and whistling. As time rolls on, the chatter intensifies. Though my grasp of Italian is basic, I understand they're in the midst of their daily lip-smacking discussion about what's for lunch. They throw ideas around with the intensity of a parliamentary debate. Should they fire up a bonfire in the old metal wheelbarrow and grill sausages, or return home to Mamma, who is making her special ragù, or just grab some panini in the village café? After much animated deliberation, they decide on the local trattoria. Why, you ask? Because it is Tuesday, of course, which means the owner will be serving his legendary homemade lasagna. As the clock strikes one, the three grown men set down their tools and skip off in the thrilling expectation of a hearty *pranzo*.

I am left smiling, quiet again, one with the world.

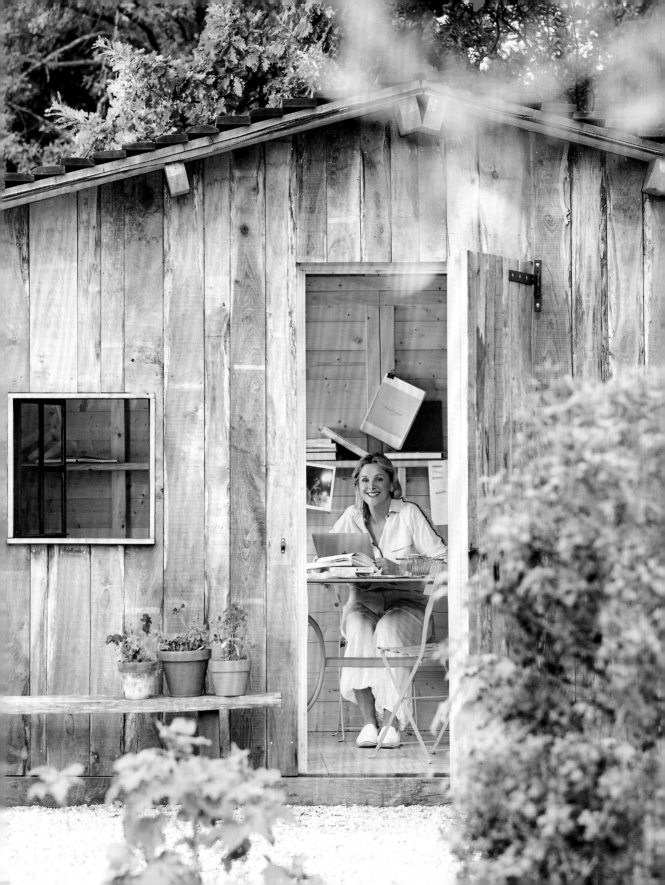

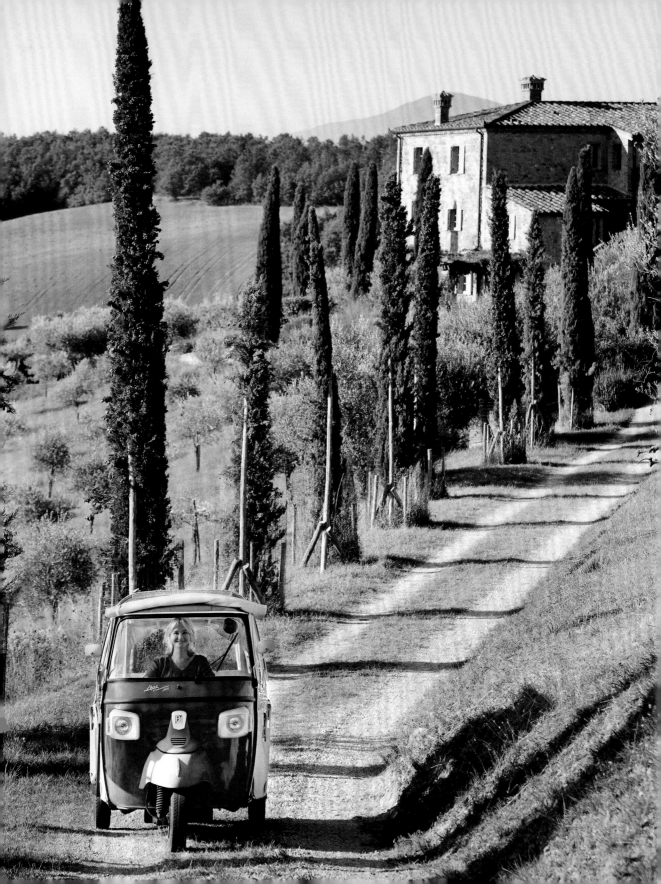

Introduction

WHAT IS IT ABOUT ITALIANS and the pure joy they have in everyday life? *La dolce vita*, the sweet life: they have turned "just being" into an art.

I have spent a lifetime crisscrossing the Atlantic Ocean. I grew up in the unpretentious confines of Northern England, but my itchy feet had me leaving home at sixteen for the hustle and bustle of London. After I met my Canadian husband, Hans, I moved across the ocean to Montreal, where I raised my children and then embarked on my television career in Canada and the United States. And now, here I am, back on the other side of the ocean, deep into my next chapter, living and running retreats in Tuscany, in the heart of Italy.

I always rooted myself deeply in the culture of each place I've called home, and I have been lucky to experience the diversity and delights of living in different countries and learning from the inhabitants of each. Nowhere is utopia, nowhere is perfect, but I have to say that when I moved to Italy, for the first time I found the path to more vitality and better balance. Even when we, as individuals, are totally committed to a healthy, joy-filled life, we're often derailed by the demands of just getting through the day. When we fall into unhealthy habits, we blame all the mess and stress the world throws at us, but we also undermine ourselves with our addiction to the toxic pace, the endless devices and the other pressures of contemporary life.

As I was writing this book, the world was hit with the novel coronavirus pandemic. The first bewildering weeks had me and almost everyone else glued to the news as it blared out updates of doom and waves of confusing and contradictory information. In shock, we did as we were told, and all of us except for essential workers stayed home to avoid contracting the virus. With nowhere to go, life was like an endless Sunday. Both worried and bored, unable to concentrate on the usual things, we dug deep into unused nesting talents. Most of us had to cook all of our meals, and some of us embraced it and discovered that we liked baking, too; once we could focus a little, we didn't just disappear into binge-watching TV—we read more, talked more, played games and reconnected with friends by phone and online. If you weren't an essential worker, if you weren't suffering financial strain, if you weren't ill, or bereaved and struggling, the excess time was a kind of gift, sprung from the chaos.

Italy was among the first countries to be hard hit. My heart sank as I wondered whether the Italian lifestyle I so treasured—with its communal closeness and multi-generational family ties—was to blame for the country's initial high rate of infection and heavy death toll. Of course it wasn't, we all realized as soon as other places came under siege and also closed their doors to neighbours, friends and family. In fact, Italian traditions and our own home countries' old ways became valuable lifelines as the pandemic tested us. Some of us met our neighbours for the first time as we began to look out for one another. I know that during lockdown I was deeply grateful for all I've learned about living from my Tuscan neighbours, and also reassured that the lessons I offer in this book will be just as crucial to creating a joy-filled life after the pandemic as they were to the life we knew before it.

Many of us have taken advantage of the unaccustomed time on our hands to analyze the way we live, to think about what matters most to us, to question how we work and what our jobs offer us, to feel our distress over what our communities value, as opposed to what they say they value or should value. We were stricken in this long crisis by the world's lack of kindness and widespread prejudice towards others as much as we were uplifted by the sacrifices of first responders, doctors, nurses and other essential workers, and devoted neighbours and volunteers. Care homes were the last place you wanted your relatives to be in the midst of the pandemic; not only has the concept of aging gracefully vanished in many places, but many countries seemed unable to provide basic care for the most vulnerable among us. The endless thirst for ever-changing technology and more new stuff has left us unmoored and spinning.

Beyond the gift of time, the other good news is that this crisis has been a giant wake-up call, showing us the cracks in the way we've been living. And I think it may

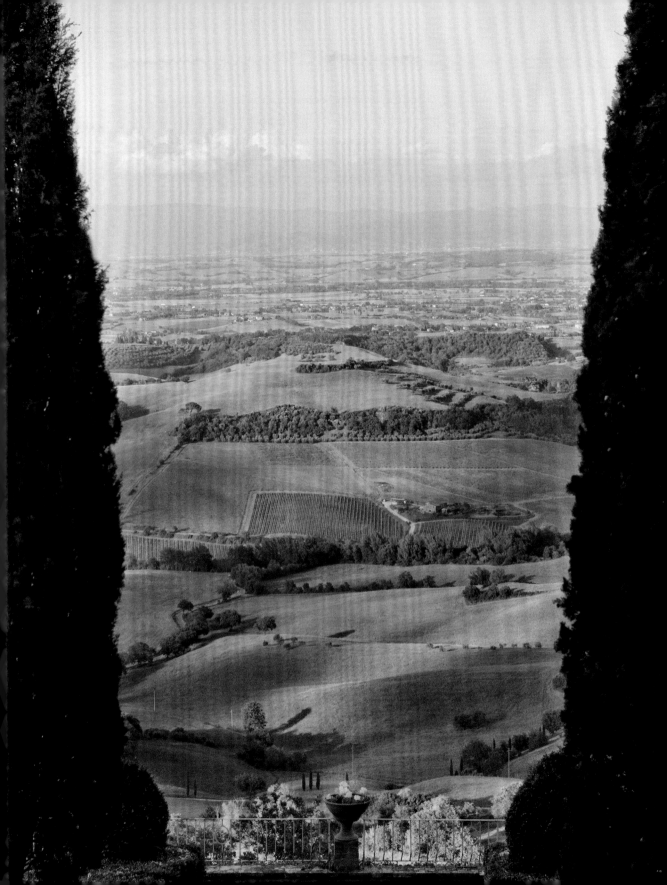

be a huge opportunity to reset and change the most unhealthy and unkind aspects of a way of life we'd been taking as "just the way things are." It has added urgency to our need to follow our dreams and move on to new horizons—which may turn out to look a lot like the ones our parents and grandparents knew, a lifestyle similar to daily life in Tuscany.

Over my years of listening to the numerous guests who visit our Tuscan retreats, I have become fully aware of their intense craving to regain their well-being, rediscover joy, increase their vitality and appreciate the simple pleasures of a balanced life. A resilient sense of purpose and meaning is so crucial if we are to live an optimal life. To unselfishly connect with a larger world beyond ourselves is good for our health and our environment. This unselfish way of living is not new. It was how past generations conducted themselves before everything became such a rush.

Movies almost always depict the Italian way of life as romantic. Much of the country is stunningly beautiful, yes—especially where I live—but it is far from perfect. Italy has high unemployment and an antiquated bureaucracy that can make doing the simplest chore laborious, but, as the novelist E.M. Forster wrote, "the people are more marvellous than the land." How true. Italy is a nation with a history of hardship and suffering, yet its people are among the healthiest and most joyful I have ever known. The Italians not only have one of the longest life expectancies in the world, but they are often blessed with an *active* old age. There is so much to learn from them.

My guests here at the villa each get a taste of wandering, without a care in the world, through a grove of olive trees bathed in Tuscan sunlight; of watching the passing scene from a café in the piazza without anything pressing to do; of sitting and staring out at the view over the valley, experiencing *la dolce far niente*: the sweetness of doing nothing. They tell me it's the simplicity of the Tuscan life that hits them in their hearts, and when it's time to leave, they always pepper me with questions about how to retain what they've experienced when they get home.

The Tuscan lifestyle is actually not that difficult to create, wherever you are, if you can reconfigure your priorities. In *JOY*, I have attempted to capture the facets of *la dolce vita* that can make every day wonderful, healthy and vital, and translate them into lessons for you to adopt to make your own life sweeter. I am not a doctor or psychiatrist or nutritionist (though you will soon meet Jacky Brown, who is an expert on healthy eating), nor do I have a magic wand to wave, but I have been lucky enough to learn from some inspiring locals. Whether you wish to hit the reset button, start a new endeavour, regain your confidence, turn a page in your relationship, make changes to your work or your community, or just reboot your vitality, I've designed each lesson in this book to help guide you to a life filled with joy.

Whoever we are, wherever we live and however old we are, it is never too late to stop and rediscover the art of living. But to do so successfully, we need to be healthy, we need to have friends, and we need a community we can rely on. We need to truly care about the issues and movements around us, educate ourselves, and find the strength and wisdom to do our part to bring about change. We require a good night's sleep and a highly nutritious diet. To spark joy in our lives again, most of us also need a sense of purpose.

With a vital body and a curious mind, we can tackle new projects undaunted and live a life brimming with energy and connection to others. We can create a lifestyle that will sustain future generations.

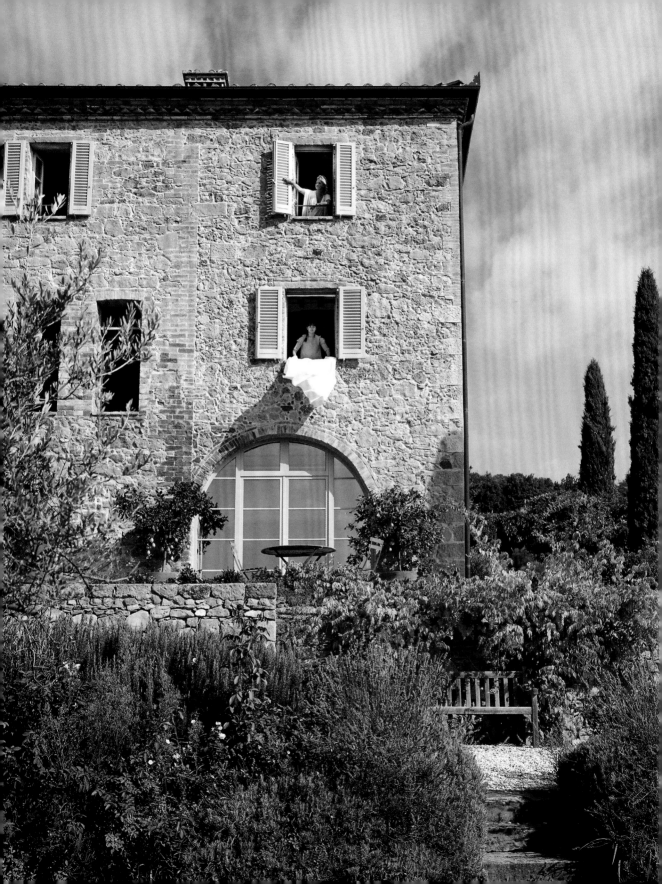

Life
at the Villa

BEFORE WE GET INTO THE PASSIONATE and powerful world of living with joy, let me describe how I recaptured my own vitality in and around Villa Reniella.

I made an enormous leap when I left the television world to run a large property in rural Tuscany. And by "run," I mean holding lifestyle retreats and farming a hundred acres of rough terrain that is home to many terraces of olive trees, where we oversee the production of two thousand bottles of extra virgin olive oil. Talk about jumping from the frying pan into the fire!

But for my own sanity, health and happiness, I had to make this big change. I've always worked hard. I've rolled up my sleeves and pulled up my socks after every disappointment, and there have been many. A strong work ethic, drive, passion and bloody-mindedness made me a success within my small world. Admirable and inspiring to others? Possibly yes, but the effort took a toll on my body, mind and soul. The constant push and pull of work and family, eating badly, glugging wine—often straight from the bottle, to unwind after a hellishly busy day—rarely finding the time to drag myself to the gym or a yoga class . . . it all left me feeling sluggish, my stress levels high and my vitality low. I tried meditation with one eye on the clock and dabbled at every diet ever invented. But you cannot trick your body into thinking you're treating it well when you're not—it always fights back. You lose sleep, you see unwelcome rolls of fat appear around your middle, and your skin becomes dull. And worse, as your sparkle in everyday life fades, you become firmly stuck in the mud.

When I first visited Italy, decades ago, I was intrigued by the differences between the life I knew and how people went about their days here. Italians work hard, and the majority are far from rich, yet everyone I met seemed to exude a sense of calm and contentment, and offered a ready smile that was immediately infectious. The ancient architecture across the country is fascinating, the food is heavenly, and the wine is *perfetto*, but it is the people and the way they conduct themselves that push us to redefine what we mean by "the good life." After every trip to Italy, I felt hooked on my own sense of renewed joy. I went back, again and again: I could not get enough of the sensibility of this country.

For ten years we sampled a variety of regions on our family vacations. We rented sprawling converted farmhouses and crumbling villas that we shared with friends and carloads of kids. These holidays were idyllic, the children running themselves ragged in unfamiliar surroundings whilst the adults relaxed in the shade, tucking into olives and bruschetta and limitless bottles of Prosecco. We lounged by pools, explored the abundant food markets and dished up meals that were uncomplicated yet deliciously varied. After each visit I felt energized, my batteries fully charged. The break from routine contributed to my sense of well-being, but there seemed to be more to it than that.

After one holiday together in Umbria (a mountainous area in the centre of Italy), a friend remarked how strange it was that she never put on weight during these jaunts. I agreed. I ate my share of pasta and never felt bloated either. Our skin glowed and our minds were crystal clear. How could this be? At home, my friends and I were terrified of pasta and bread. Wine was a guilty pleasure, and relaxing and chatting with friends into the wee hours—well, who had time for that?

Eventually, Hans and I decided we needed to make a home here. We put pins in the map and set off on expeditions that took us from the foothills of the Alps in the

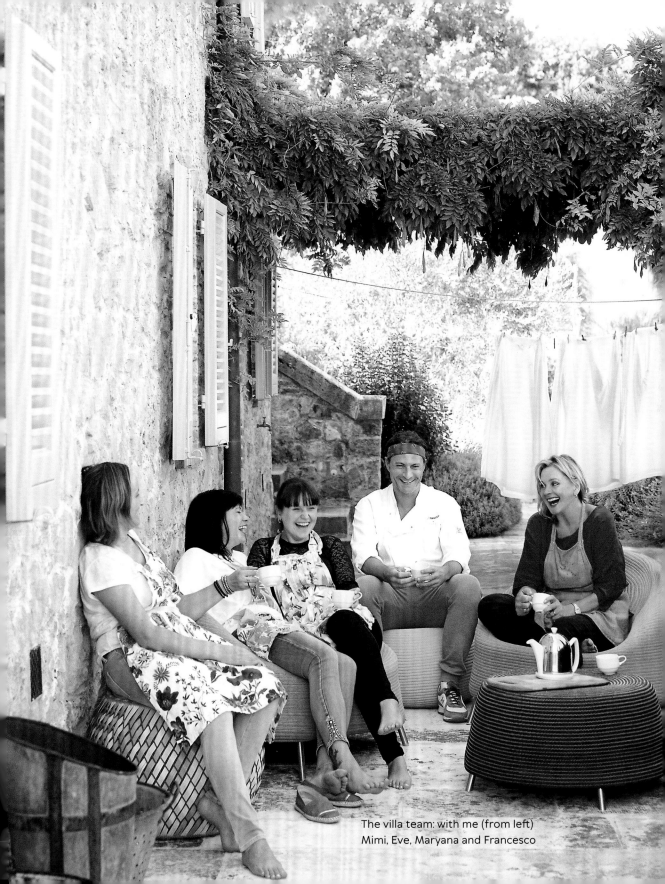

The villa team: with me (from left)
Mimi, Eve, Maryana and Francesco

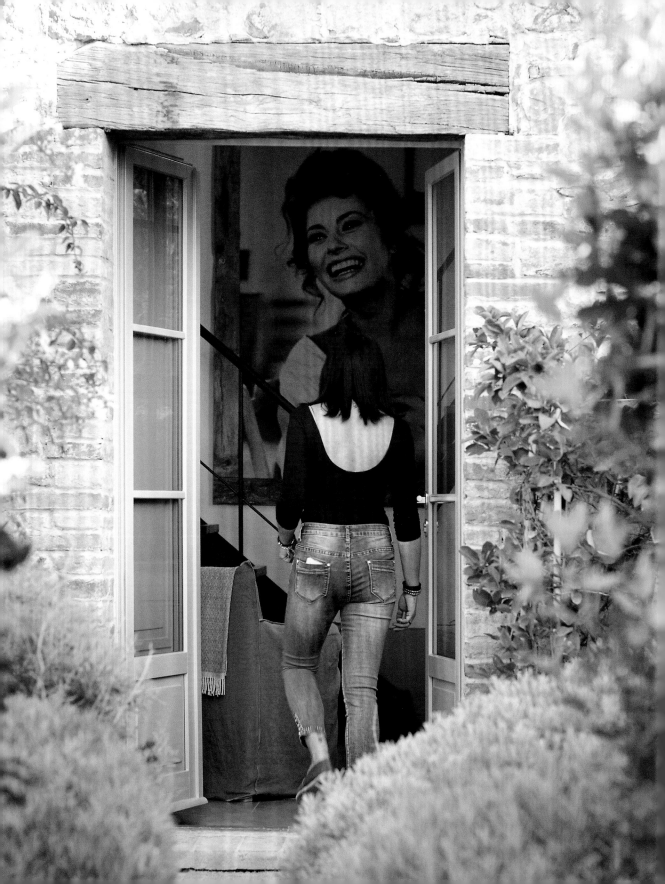

north to the Sicilian beaches at the end of the Italian boot. But our search soon narrowed to one particular valley between the quintessential Tuscan towns of Pienza and Montepulciano; that's where the true meaning of this sweet, vital life began to truly resonate for us.

After months of searching for a property that ticked all the boxes, we homed in on a particular area. And at the end of a day's search, we came across a bar jammed with locals below the medieval gates of the thirteenth-century village of Montefollonico. The sun was setting as we quietly fell into the evening ritual of the *aperitivo*—drinks and a spread of small snacks for the patrons to munch on. On this first visit, the barista was pleasant to us strangers, but the second time we went, he greeted us with such delight and enthusiasm that we were convinced he had mistaken us for long-lost cousins. The third time we dropped by (in as many days), we were rewarded with complimentary biscotti alongside a small glass of something both sweet and fierce. On all our future visits, the locals offered us welcoming smiles as we took our seats in the piazza, and Tomas, the barista, would straddle a chair beside us for an animated chat. It was strange to us anglophones, but we felt accepted by the people of the valley.

One evening, downtrodden and defeated from our endless searching, we dropped by for a much-needed Campari. After serving the drinks, Tomas sat down and asked why we looked so sad. We explained that we were having no luck with our hunt for a home in Tuscany. His reaction amazed us. Throwing his arms in the air, he listed several homes that he knew were for sale through the never-ending gossip he heard in the café. He then pointed to a couple of old men, members of a large family who had owned a nearby farm for many generations. They had sold the property a few years before to foreigners who had now decided they wished to sell. Tables were thrown together and introductions made. More drinks were ordered for all as the gentlemen described the property. It had been a poor working farm in their day and was still a partial ruin. The two men promised to set up a visit for the next day. That night, we lay awake in our lodgings. Had we stumbled upon our future home?

It turned out that, yes, we had. Though in some ways the place wasn't exactly the dream situation I had imagined. Parts of the five-hundred-year-old farmhouse had been modernized—in 1950, when the first inside kitchen had been installed. There was only one bathroom in the entire place, and the animals—at least, the four pigs that remained—still lived happily in the dirt on the ground floor. But disappointment turned to elation as we looked out at the view. Piggies aside, we had found our beloved Villa Reniella.

After buying the property, it dawned on us that owning our own Italian home wasn't a big enough dream. We needed to share this corner of paradise with others, even strangers. With much hard work to achieve our oversized visions, we turned Villa Reniella into not only our home but a retreat centre where guests could experience the delights of Tuscan living first-hand and take home the tools to boost their vitality and purpose.

What still blows our minds is the exuberance and energy we feel whenever we spend time at the villa and in the surrounding villages. *Alive* is the simplest way to describe it. There is a spring in our step, a persistent joy in our hearts, and we smile more. Every time, it's like rolling into the gas station on empty, then surging back onto the road with a full tank, heading to new horizons.

With this book, I want to spread Tuscan wisdom and its gift of joy and renewal even further, so that you will be energized to feel what we feel, even if you never leave home.

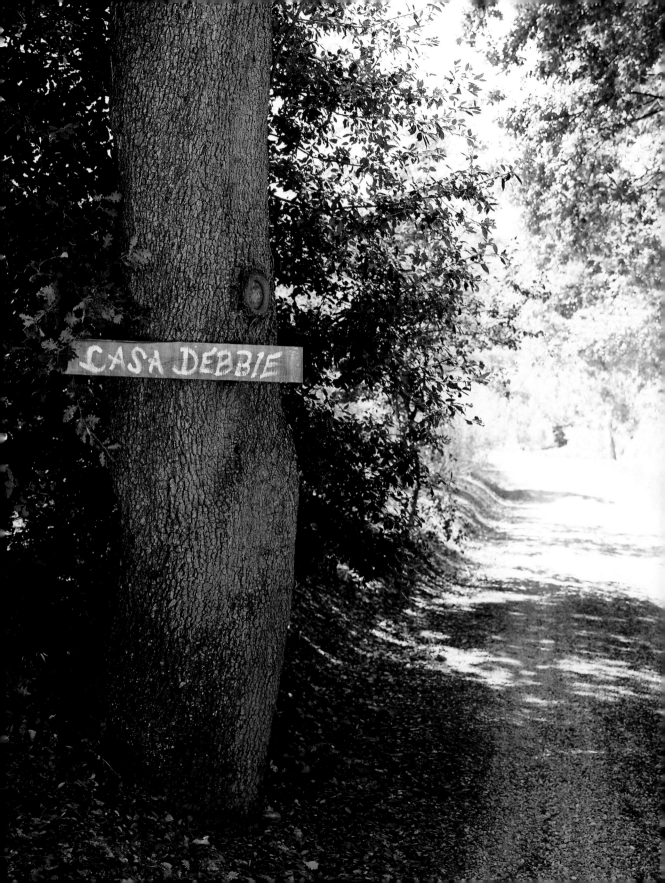

What Is Vitality, Where Did It Go and How Do We Get It Back?

MOST OF US DON'T THINK ABOUT our vitality until it's gone. And then we're faced with a real challenge: how do we get it back?

We may lose vitality in a steady trickle over time, or we may come to a sudden realization that our mojo has dried up. Diminished energy, finding endless excuses to stay static and an inability to hatch future plans are all signs that we have lost our sense of self, our fullness, our joy. First we need to be reintroduced to our vital self, and then we can build vitality back into our daily life.

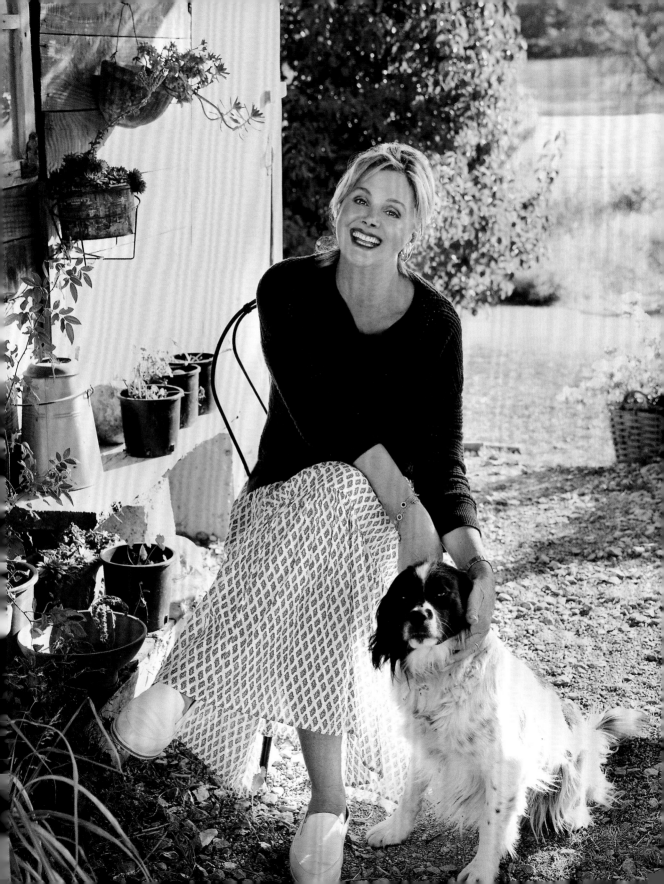

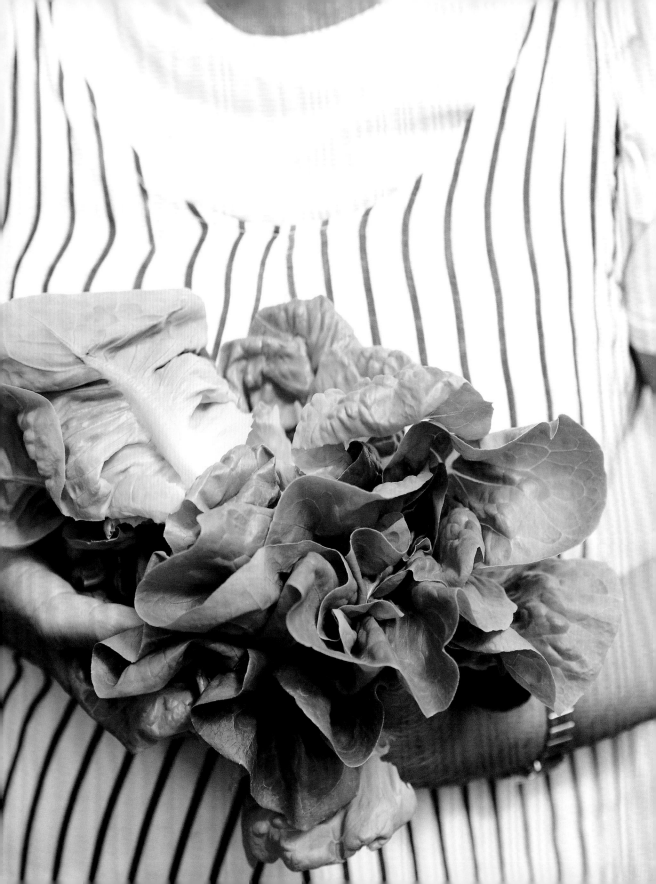

Vita, the Latin root of *vitality*, means "life." Most languages have a term for this internal energy, the living force that lies inside us. In France it is *raison d'être*—a reason for being. The concept of vitality is engrained in Eastern philosophies and is the core of their traditional healings. The Chinese believe in *qi* (ch'i), or energy flow. The Indian notion of *prana* is about finding the energy source through breathing. In Bali, vitality is called *bayu*, and in Japan, it is *ki*—energy released.

In the modern world, increased stress and the pace of life can crush our energy levels. Vitality is a positive energy that is awarded to us in its natural form; it is not an energy boost fuelled by caffeine, alcohol or sugary treats.

We enter this world kicking and screaming, with a stubborn determination to survive. We begin life's journey as vital human beings, and some of us manage to take our vitality from cradle to grave. You know who I mean: those people who seem to exude an aura of energy, like they are naturally backlit. A glint in the eye, an easy laugh, a magnetic force. Those with vitality have an infectious get-up-and-go attitude that draws others to them. Most of us, though, don't experience vitality as an inexhaustible force; we have ups and downs, and if we don't watch it, the downs gradually grow longer than the ups, as life becomes messy and complicated.

But it is challenging to step out of the shadows—to begin a new project, develop new friends or work to hang on to old ones—if we allow our vital life force to fade away. And even though our vitality has deep roots, as a tree of life that is constantly growing, blooming and sending out tendrils and branches into the universe, it needs to be tended. A period of stillness, rest and rejuvenation, better food for our bodies, connection to others to warm our souls, meaningful work to get us up in the morning: all of these things help restore our zest for living and curiosity about the world. In essence, living a vital life is simply about waking up looking forward to the day ahead and falling asleep at night content that your day has had meaning and value.

Some of my guests at the villa visit simply because Tuscany is on their bucket list. But many others come looking for rejuvenation of all kinds, including renewed vitality. They ache for even a sliver of the spirit of their younger, more energetic selves.

And this is a gift we can share, because Tuscan life has vitality at its very heart. At the retreats, we hike and bike together through landscapes so beautiful they leave us breathless. We share endless stories over glasses of wine and partake in the two-hour-long communal meals that are synonymous with the Tuscan lifestyle—food for the soul, the body and the heart. Wooden tables under the olive trees are laden with vases of wildflowers and boundless dishes of traditional Tuscan fare. Plates piled with crostini of melted pecorino cheese, pear and truffle oil, salads from the garden tossed with toasted chickpeas. Mountains of steamed vegetables slathered in olive oil and roasted garlic, slices of succulent pork, ravioli stuffed with puréed artichoke, and copious bottles of chilled wine . . . Should I go on? Are you drooling?

These are romantic images of the perfect holiday, but the much larger truth beneath the fairy-tale vision comes from the face-to-face conversations. Groups of all ages and backgrounds open up to strangers in this non-judgmental environment, where they can take the time to marvel not at their differences, but at how much alike they are. It is impossible for even the most reserved person to resist the camaraderie of a long, leisurely Tuscan lunch. As the days unfold, we watch as our guests' vitality bubbles to the surface again, shining from each beaming face.

Following the publication of my last book, *Design Your Next Chapter*, I heard from thousands of readers, by e-mail and on social media, who wished to share their stories. They fell into two rough categories. The first were those who joyfully told me about their journey into new experiences, how they had turned the page to follow their dream. Some had packed in the corporate world to start a fresh venture; others had gone back to school or taken up travel, or even moved to another country or taken on rural living. Thankfully, not one of them told me they regretted their decision.

The people in the other category broke my heart. They wanted me to know that they had found it impossible to explore new outlets or make any form of improvement because they couldn't tap the passion, strength and fervour required to move forward. They felt so numbed and unconfident, they couldn't even dream. The biggest shocker was that these communications weren't just from older people who felt too worn out by their struggles to change how they were living, but also from people in their twenties. If you are at the younger end of the age spectrum and you feel that life is a drag, find little that motivates you and have realized that your best friend is an Instagram account, then you, too, need to take action.

I find it impossible to feel jaded when I sit in a particular piazza in Rome, taking in my surroundings. If I had to define vitality, it would be what I see right here: a balance of time standing still and people living with energy. It is the heartfelt conversation between the couple three tables away; the animated waiter passionately describing the dish of the day in mouth-watering detail; the tourist whose smile turns dreamy as she gazes over the square, knowing she will relive this moment for many years to come. Here is life lived with balance and joy.

Vitality has little to do with age. Giulia, a centenarian living in our village, recently started a new business. To help raise money for the local primary school, she opened the tiniest of shops, selling donated bric-a-brac. Her speciality is over-starched pairs of antique lace knickers, perhaps even her own from a bygone era. I am not sure she is doing a roaring trade, but there she sits on her tatty wicker chair, on the days she chooses to open, chatting with every passerby. Her good health, even at her very ripe old age, gives her the vitality to run her shop, which in turn brings her and others joy.

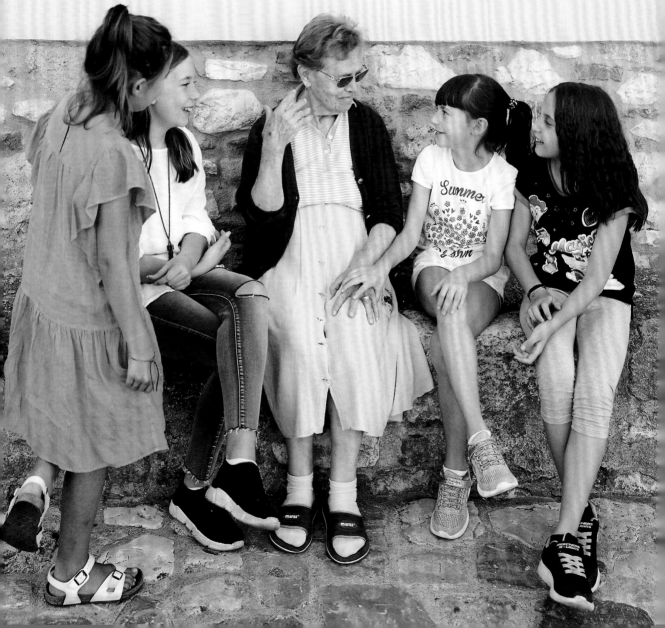

Longevity Is Not Just About Living Longer

MY LITTLE TUSCAN VILLAGE is ruled by octogenarians, still productive and vital in old age. At the supermarket, there is always a chair by the bread counter where a town elder will park themselves for a chat. There is often a painfully long wait at the teeny bank, which is the size of your average suburban bathroom, as you find yourself behind a sprightly retiree regaling the patient bank clerk with the wonders of their great-grandchildren or yesterday's pasta triumph. It's an absolute no-no to try to hurry them along.

Each day at the bar, weather permitting, old ladies plonk themselves down on plastic chairs in lively groups, or perch on the low walls like impatient flocks of birds, and chatter away. You may even find the odd teenager sandwiched in between a couple of *nonnas*. Men of all ages also gather here from sun-up, all offering hearty "*Buongiornos*" as they down a quick grappa slipped into their first espresso of the day. When the working men have departed on tractors, in vans or in Ferraris, the old men carry on with the gossip and political discussions until whatever chore they have for the day calls, then pick up where they left off that evening, during the *aperitivo* hour. Sometimes I think the main secret to their longevity is that they are people who take the time to enjoy other people.

Most of us wish for longevity, but on our own terms. No one relishes the thought of spending their last days rattling pill bottles, just passing time, possibly alone. For some, that fate is unavoidable, but the rest of us owe it to ourselves to give a better life our best shot. You cannot have longevity unless you have vitality, good health, an active mind and days filled with joy. So many of us are afraid of becoming elderly that at every age we proclaim we are not yet old. "Sixty is the new forty," and so on. But the important thing, I've learned, is not the years etched on our faces but our quality of life.

Longevity is a topic so attention-grabbing that scientists from around the world study it in places called Blue Zones: countries such as Italy, Japan, Costa Rica and Greece, as well as one particular area of California, where the populations are the longest-living on the planet. Dan Buettner, author of *The Blue Zones: Lessons for Living Longer from the People Who've Lived the Longest*, has travelled with his team to discover the secrets of these communities, including a small hilltop area in Sardinia, an island off the coast of Italy where the population is the longest-living in the world. According to the World Health Organization, Italy is consistently within the top three countries for overall health and longevity, and Sardinia has ten times more centenarians per capita than North America. Genes play a role, of course, but Dr. Gianni Pes, an Italian scientist who collected the first data on the long lives of the Sardinians, found that longevity isn't due to any one element. Factors that play a role include eating well, drinking alcohol in moderation, getting enough exercise and being part of a community—feeling like you are valued and not just a burden.

Adapting to the rhythm of the Tuscan lifestyle has given me a taste of pure joy and rebooted my vitality. Living here has shown me the ways in which *la dolce vita* safeguards vitality and encourages longevity. But it has also reminded me that my parents and grandparents knew the importance of these lessons too. Perhaps the biggest lesson I've learned is that the best way forward sometimes leans heavily on the wisdom of the past.

ADELINA

Adelina sits in her favourite chair in the hair salon we both frequent, holding court like the queen she is, sharing gossip and thriving on the stories she tells and hears. When her white hair is perfectly coiffed, she moves to a chair outside the door and carries on chatting with those around her. Well into her nineties, she is as elegant and beautiful as a delicate bird. The street she lives on is her entire world. One day, I told her she was *bellissima*, and with a devilish look in her eye, she replied, "I was once the prettiest girl in town, but sadly not anymore." As I was about to vehemently disagree, she announced with a giggle, "But I do have a date tonight." True vitality, even into her tenth decade.

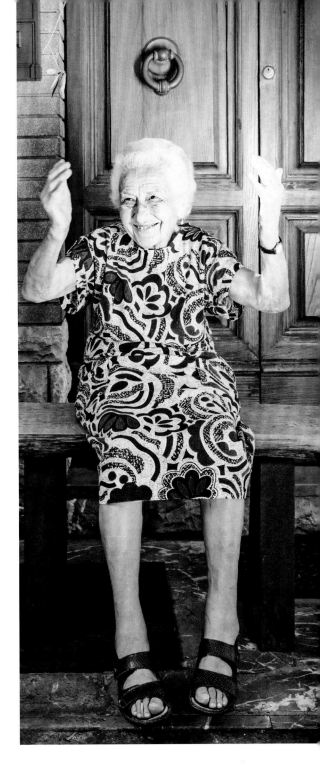

Meet Jacky Brown, Nutritional Therapist

I NEVER IMAGINED THAT I WOULD write a book about health, vitality and longevity. I have no expertise in this area—far from it, given my meagre high-school education. I can see with my own eyes (and feel in my own body) the health benefits of the Tuscan lifestyle. But to offer you the best advice on the health benefits of the Tuscan way of eating and drinking, I needed expert help, so I recruited Jacky Brown, my oldest and dearest friend, to be the professional voice behind the lessons in this book.

When I began to dream of opening a small hotel in Tuscany where we would hold retreats, Jacky and her husband, Steve, joined with Hans and me to make it come true. Our first retreat, which took place in a rented villa in 2009, was an immediate success. It was so unexpected. We knew that bringing a group of women together to have fun under the Tuscan sun was a great idea, but it materialized into so much more than a memorable vacation. Jacky and I looked on, flabbergasted, as our guests for the week transformed before our eyes. Personalities became brighter, stomachs flatter, eyes shinier and smiles broader. Was it just the large amount of wine we were consuming, or was there something else going on?

Jacky and I began to dig deeper. We researched everything we could find on longevity, levels of heart disease, cancer and obesity, and the lifestyles of people in different areas of Italy. We were fascinated to discover how the findings here compared to those in North America and the United Kingdom. More proof of the potential health benefits of the Tuscan lifestyle was only a five-minute walk away, with the population of the local village.

Jacky soon decided she had to take her knowledge about the intriguing subject of an optimal lifestyle to the next level. She left her job as the chief financial officer of a construction company and, in her early fifties, went back to school. This was daunting, to say the least: in a class of forty-eight students, she was the oldest by an average of twenty years. Fast-forward a few years. Jacky graduated from London's College of Naturopathic Medicine and is now a member of the British Association

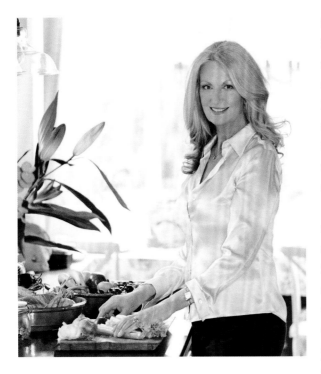

for Nutrition and Lifestyle Medicine, DipCMM, mBANT. She was one of only six students who lasted through the whole course, and she now has her own practice and leads the nutritional way on our retreats.

Naturopathic nutritionists, such as Jacky, advocate preventing illness and promoting self-healing of the body through a diverse and varied diet, natural therapies and an active lifestyle. They believe optimal nutrition is the foundation of a healthy mind and body. They understand that all the systems of the body are interconnected, and if one element is out of balance, it may affect the others. Jacky treats the whole person, not the disease, searching out the root or underlying causes of an illness, not just the symptoms. Her approach is founded on empathy and the belief that we are all individuals with different needs.

There is an abundance of conflicting health advice in the media today that has left many of us bewildered, so I wanted to make sure that the lessons in this book are supported by the best science-backed research and information available to us at the time of writing. "Jacky says . . ." is a phrase that often comes out of my mouth when I'm explaining healthy living to guests and friends. And I'm relying on Jacky to help us make sense of it all here, too!

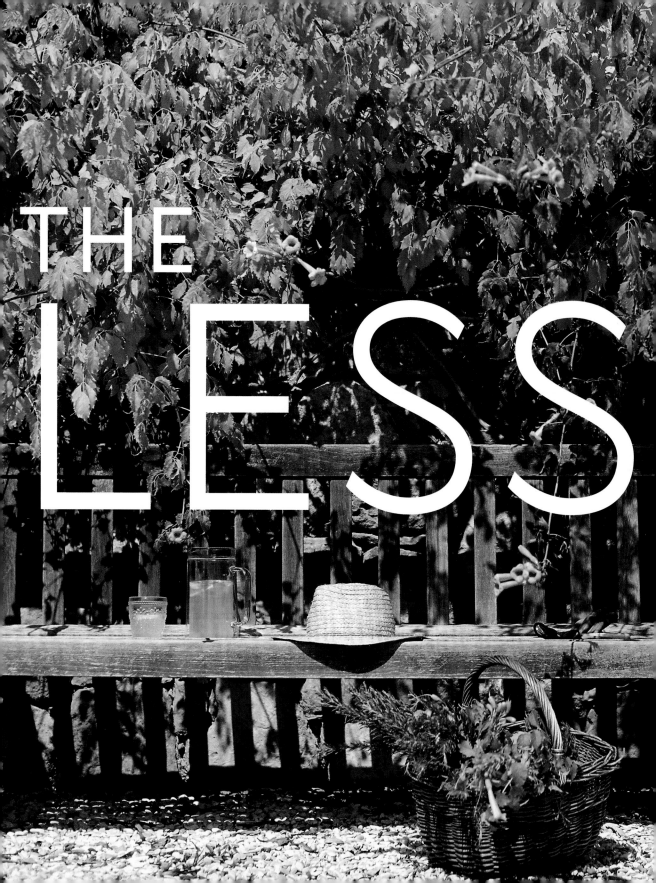

THE
LESS

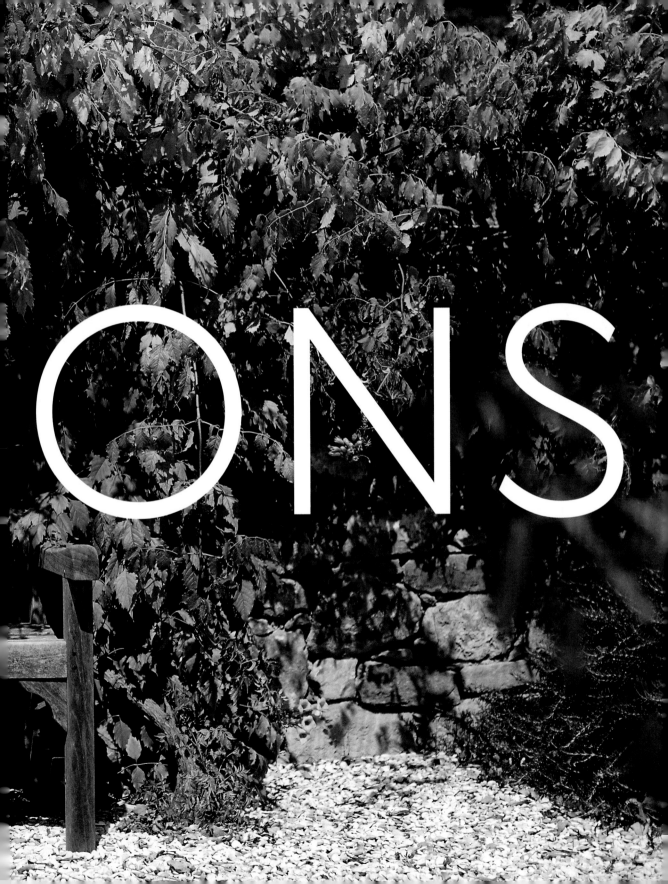

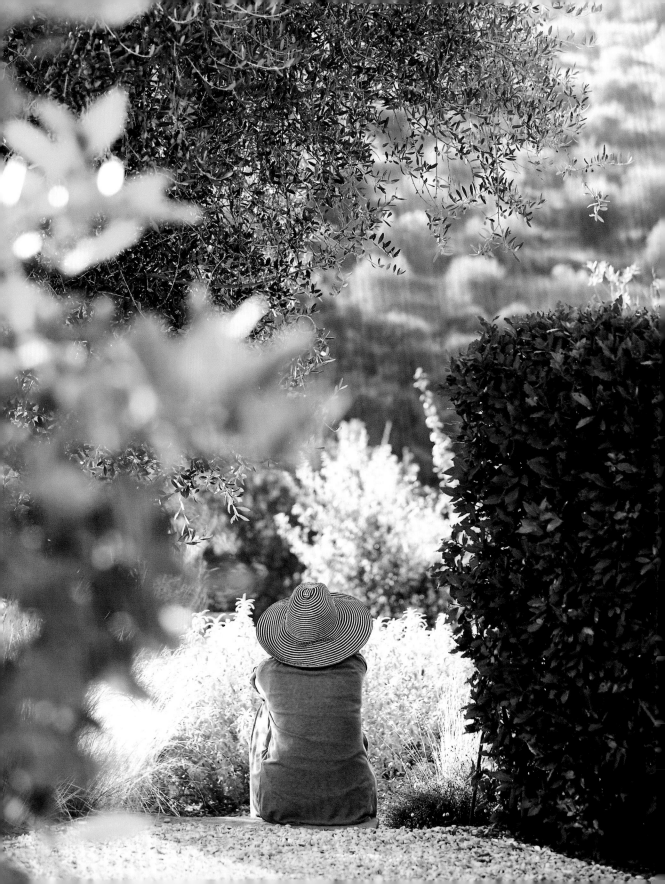

Realize
Reset
Restore
Revitalize

OUR LIVES MIRROR THE JOURNEY OF A RIVER—never straight, never predictable. A river may be lazy and meandering at times, then turn into a torrent of whitewater over wild rocks or even drop over a cliff in a spectacular, terrifying waterfall. But while a river can seem to flow with no intention or purpose, and can even descend into chaos, it always finds its way in the end to the welcoming lake or the open sea. Our emotions, too, are rarely still. Given our nature and the twists in the river of our lives, it is unrealistic to strive for a steady current of happiness. But we can all aim, at least, to find more joy.

In a way, you can blame this book on my last one, *Design Your Next Chapter*, in which I shared my story—why I decided to make such a radical change to pursue my Tuscan dream, even though, to most people, my life seemed like it was already a wild success—along with similar stories from other people. Time and again, readers reached out to tell me that they, too, wanted to find a new life and follow a dream, but they just didn't have the energy to do so. They had the need, but not the vitality. So many of us feel ground down by the things we think we have to do to pay the rent, succeed at work and raise our kids, but we also get caught up in the endless quest for more and better—a bigger house, the perfect partner, the ultimate diet, the fountain of youth. But human happiness and vitality springs from a much simpler source than working ourselves into the ground in order to have the best of everything—which is something I've learned here in Tuscany.

Every time we return to the villa, it only takes a handful of days to begin to see change in ourselves. Our guests, most of whom are here for only a week, are gobsmacked at the difference in how they feel when they wake up in the morning. It's difficult to explain, but picture that pleasant feeling you get when a child waves at you for no reason from a car window on the highway. You smile and wave back, appreciating the instant jolt of warmth you receive from that child's innocent gesture. For a precious moment, you feel full of hope and are stress-free. You feel a similar little charge when a friend gives you a hug for just being you, or when the stranger you've just chatted with in the café buys you a coffee. Or maybe you are that stranger, reaching out. It feels good, doesn't it? The life I've discovered and that we've created here in Tuscany is about a series of such moments of connection, bolstered by a deep appreciation that humans need kinship and meaning to feel good about themselves and the world.

The following ten lessons spring from what I have learned from the Italian culture, and especially from life in rural Tuscany. While we can't all go live in a village on a hillside covered in olive groves, we can make simple changes in our lives that bring that Tuscan feeling home. But first we need to recognize the state we're in now, reset the parameters of what's important in our life and restore our health and energy. Then and only then will we feel revitalized and ready to move forward—and even to create our next chapter!

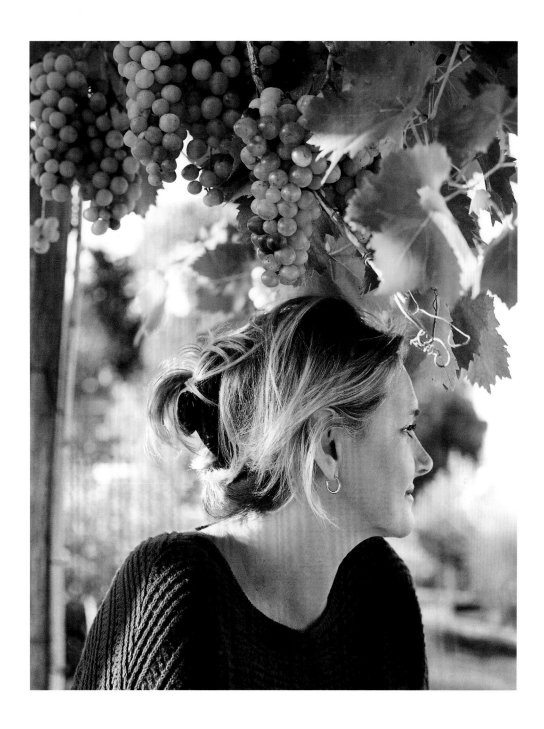

REALIZE RESET RESTORE REVITALIZE

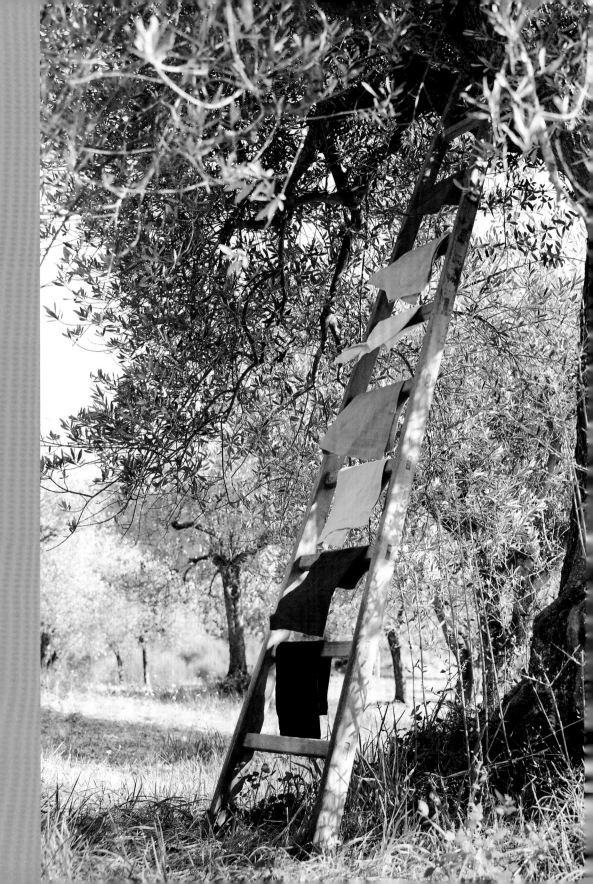

The JOY Ladder

WHEN THE VILLA WAS UNDER CONSTRUCTION and I had to rough it in the rubble, I used a wooden olive-picking ladder to dry my clothes. I would prop it against the branches of the hardy old olive trees, thinking about how they have survived centuries of wars, famine and heartbreak, but have also witnessed scenes of joy as they delivered their bounty to so many generations. While I was pondering a way to visually represent how people could reset themselves on their journey towards joy, I thought of my old ladder, hung this time with napkins whose colours represent the way you feel, from dark days to vibrant happiness:

■ PITCH BLACK

Everyone drops into this joyless place from time to time, and heartbreak and trauma can cause us to pay more extended visits to the dark zone. If you lock those sad, angry, fearful feelings away, they will fester and intensify and leave you trapped here. If this is your steady state, reach out for help.

■ MIDNIGHT BLUE

Perched on this indigo-coloured rung, we may find ourselves not exactly depressed but feeling emotionally low. We become irritated by the routines of daily life and snap easily. We often seek isolation, thinking we need to be alone. We all feel the midnight blues at times, but it is not a place we wish to hang around for long.

■ GREEN

Green is a transitional stage, one that can symbolize new beginnings. Here we find ourselves more calm and grounded than on the bottom two rungs of the ladder. Maybe it's best described as neither here nor there: we're not in distress—we're fully capable of getting through the day—but we're not exactly ablaze with energy and inspiration. It's fine to be green, but events and issues can quickly upset your equilibrium, pushing you back to one of the lower rungs. Classic imagery paints jealousy and envy as green; giving in to either will quickly drop you down a rung or two.

■ AQUAMARINE

To me, this foamy turquoise colour, a blend of blue and yellow, signifies stasis. If someone were to ask you how you were feeling when you were in this state, you'd likely reply, "Just fine, thank you." But fine is all you'd be. And saying "fine" is one step away from apathy. On this rung, you need to dig deep to unearth more purpose; when you do, you'll notice the difference between being fine and feeling vital.

■ PEACEFUL YELLOW

There is nothing quite like the sun coming up in the morning. With the sun on our face, we dream of forever possibilities. The feeling of the yellow zone is unique to each individual. Many are focused and engaged, bathing themselves in the sunny spotlight. For others, yellow's intense energy can be overwhelming, like being stuck in a room with banana-coloured walls. If your yellow zone evokes an edgy aggressiveness rather than the serenity of a sunflower, reset your balance by dipping into the quiet aqua below, then reach up for the glowing rungs above.

■ SWEET ORANGE

Grabbing the orange rung snaps us into the vitality zone. We become increasingly generous, kinder to others and motivated. Our sense of joy is contagious, and we love to spread it to our friends, family and community. This is a sweet place to be, for sure, but it is unrealistic to imagine ourselves staying here forever. It is normal to drop frequently to the rungs below, but the key is to strive to return to the orange rung.

■ RICH RED

It is precarious at the top of the ladder. Though we have to be in the right mood to wear bright red lipstick or a flaming red tie, we own our world when we do. It would be exhausting to stay here too long; balance is the key to a well-lived life. To be as bold as a red sports car is not for everyone, but we all deserve to dip in and out of the red zone. Reaching for more joy is a thrill, whatever our age.

HOW TO USE THE JOY LADDER

One of the most interesting things I've learned from working with the people who come on the retreats is how often we don't really know how we're feeling. A crucial part of learning to live a life with more joy is understanding what makes you feel good and what brings you down. So grab a bunch of crayons and pin up a calendar where you will see it every day. Over the course of a month, colour in each day—or even different parts of each day—with the colour from the ladder that best reflects your mood. For the next month, keep on filling in your mood calendar every day, but now also record the situations that trigger a particular mood. You will likely see a pattern forming.

Nobody lives in the sunny shades all the time, and all of us will dive down into the blues and the blacks. But the calendar will reveal how long you stay in those darker colours and help you find ways to plug all your energy leaks and climb towards a more vital life.

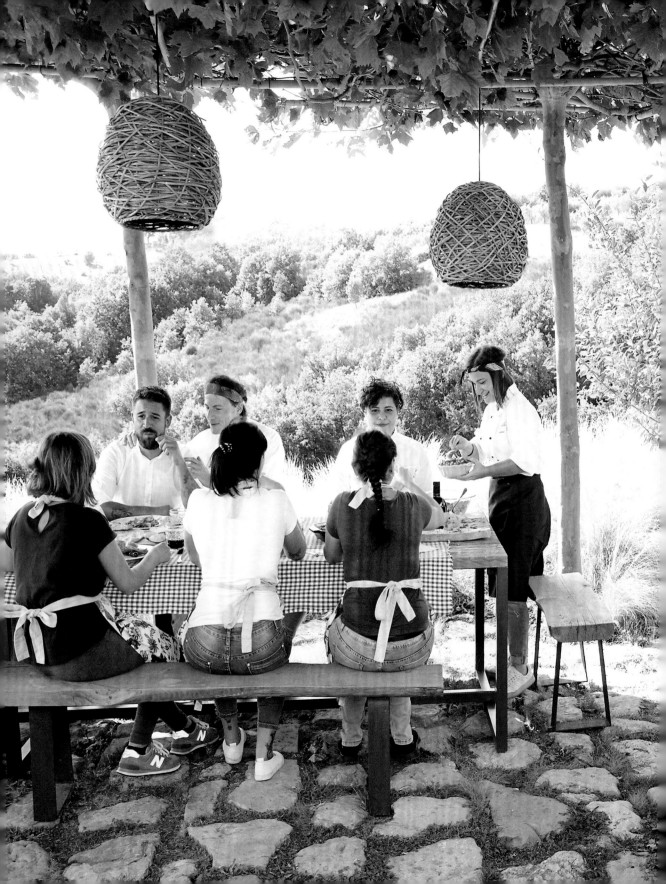

Build Your Community

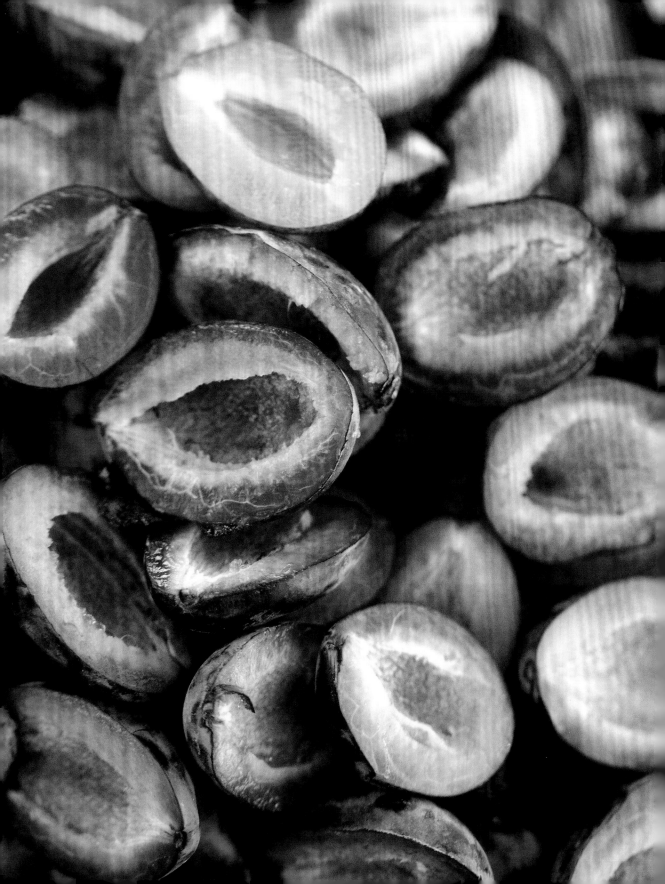

Born to Unite

IT IS UNCANNY HOW SIMILAR one aspect of my childhood in Northern England is to the life I lead now at Villa Reniella. Neighbours!

We kids recognized all the faces of the people who came together at village get-togethers, jumble sales in the school hall and around my mum's kitchen table. We knew their relatives, their life circumstances, when they needed help and who to go to when we needed help. It was a place in which people knew how to ease each other's suffering through kindness and community action.

Strong communities like the one where I grew up are a life force. When I was a kid, they were more the norm rather than the exception. But it's no wonder so many of us feel lonely and isolated now, given how many forces are undermining our communities. City high-rises with few communal spaces have replaced neighbourhoods with front stoops and backyard fences, and in many families, all of the adults now have to work to pay the bills, commuting instead of spending time getting to know their neighbours. Our material lives may have improved over the last decades, but at what cost?

Like so many young people then (and today), I could not wait to leave the confines of village life and head for the big-city lights and my own dreams. What teenager wants their family and all their neighbours, no matter how loving, watching their every move! But I am glad to have come full circle. I cannot tell you the comfort I find in being back once more in a place where I know my neighbours, in a country where there is plenty of sophistication and urban glamour a short drive away, but also such respect for the kind of communal living that touches something deep in the human soul.

Here at our villa—which was, for generations before us, the Trombetti farm, or *podere*—about twenty members of the same family once lived in these stone-floored rooms with their soaring arched ceilings, over the pigs, chickens and cattle stabled below. Though they eventually sold up and moved into a brand-new building with all the mod-cons in the village, like many Italian families, especially in Tuscany, they still live together—the grandparents on one floor, the married children and grandchildren on another, and the singles in their own quarters.

The thought of having your parents living upstairs, or even around the corner from you, may sound like hell on earth. I can hear my own children screaming, "Not a chance, Mum and Dad! You are *NOT* moving in with us—we're planning to send you to the Windy Pines Assisted Living Centre." Very funny, but as I keep explaining to them, there are countless benefits when families (or even groups of friends) live under one roof. Younger generations can keep a watchful eye on the elderly; babysitters are built-in; and if parents are working out of the home, there are more people to do school pickups and prepare meals. Most importantly, in such a set-up, it's very hard to be lonely!

While this lifestyle mostly vanished in North America and much of Europe in the last half of the twentieth century, in our current economic era, with real estate prices through the roof, first-time homeowners having a tough time getting a foothold in the market, and people in their twenties and thirties boomeranging home as they try to get established in the world, there is a financial incentive to share households. As the recognition of the benefits of face-to-face relationships grows, we are seeing families (and groups of friends) choosing to upsize to larger properties they can share with their parents, grown kids and children. Everything old is new again!

Living together, or at least regularly gathering together, is important to everyone. Not only do we find emotional well-being in our face-to-face relationships, but seeing others on a regular basis has a positive physical effect on us as well. Research tells us that people who regularly engage with others in a social setting feel less stress and are healthier, less obese and less vulnerable to infectious diseases, including the common cold.

In the town where I grew up, there were lots of regular events and annual celebrations. In Italy, where rural villages were often isolated because it was so challenging to get around, the residents organized their own local entertainment. These days, most people have access to modern transport, but the traditional events—a different festival just about every week, it seems—are still popular.

In our village there's fish night in the piazza once a month and a *Buona Festa dei Nonni*: a celebration of the local grandparents. The *vendemmia*—the picking of the grapes— is a not-to-be-missed opportunity to gather in the vineyards. A few weeks later, we celebrate the olive harvest. Then there are the regular street parties, with hundreds from the village and the nearby countryside tucking into vast meals on tables that snake their way down the main street. Tents are erected in those same streets for a whole weekend in December for the Vin Santo festival, an excuse to indulge in free samples of this sweet local wine. In March, certain rural areas hold their own *palio*— not the world-famous horse race that takes place annually in the centre of Siena, but a more low-key affair where enthusiastic riders race donkeys around the town parking lot. Our plumber has won our local *palio* for the last ten years!

Though we are expats, my husband and I feel folded into the life of our village in a way that truly brings joy. And the fact that so many people these days live an individualistic life, lacking relationships and community, is brought home to me with every retreat. When our guests arrive, we give them a handmade leather-bound diary and encourage them to jot down reflections, dreams and ways to bring more joy into their lives. By the end of the week, every single person has written something in their diary about how they long to bring a sense of community home with them.

How to Find Your Tribe

The reality is that most of us don't live in quaint small towns with a long tradition of looking out for each other and celebrating together. Instead, we have to work to replace the old ways of meeting people with new ones, building a fresh version of community. Imagine if you could meet fifty new people a year—the odds are that one of them would become a confidant, a true friend. I really had to figure out how to meet people and develop a social life when we moved to Tuscany, with the extra hurdle of the language barrier; I have no gift for languages, and my Italian is still rudimentary after ten years! My solution was to seek out the many expats with homes and businesses in the area.

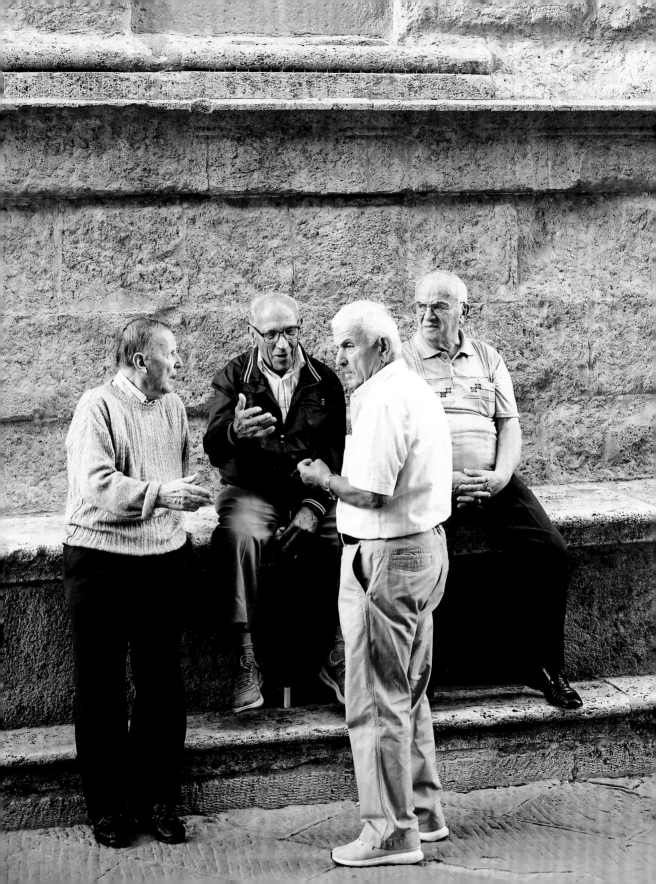

Our place is a constant whirlwind of casual lunches and *aperitivos*, which are all about human contact! It costs so little to throw together a sliced baguette with a variety of scrumptious toppings—or crostini, as the Italians call it. Add a bowl of olives and a bunch of crispy radishes, and you have all you need for a get-together. I offer such invitations all the time to strangers. Some turn out not to be my type, but I have found many interesting new friends this way.

Release yourself from the confinement of another evening alone and ask an acquaintance or three to pop by for a drink. You'll be surprised by how rarely such an invitation is refused. Invite a neighbour who is also often alone. Take the lead from the never-ending social life of the Tuscans and make a habit of having friends around on a regular basis. It is an all-win situation.

Be a Joiner

My old friend Barb moved away from Toronto, where she was deeply connected to her community, to be near her sister, who lived in a rural town a hundred kilometres away. Barb was in her forties and needed to be part of things, but found it daunting to start building a social life all over again. After two weeks of crying and feeling desperately sorry for herself, she joined just about everything going: the local drama group, the church choir, the Sunday morning hikers and even the knitting circle. She didn't take to the drama club, and she realized she could not sing and was all thumbs when it came to knitting, but the hiking stuck and she especially enjoyed the group visits to the café after the walk was over. Here she was able to make friends with new people she enjoyed.

Simple, I know, but join things! If you don't like one activity, try something else. We are more likely to connect with others over a shared interest, whether that's working, exercising, eating or sipping wine together. If you normally head to the gym after work, try gathering some people to go for a drink and a laugh afterwards. It will have as big an impact on your well-being as sweating it out in the gym.

Sharing a meal with people is a wonderful way to reinforce your relationships and find new friends; preparing food together may be an even better way, as many neighbourhoods are learning with the advent of community kitchens in which old and new community members get together and share their recipes, along with their culture.

I remember how my mother and her friends would gather and turn a chore—preserving the abundance of a summer harvest—into an excuse for laughter and conversation as they created jars of what seemed like every jam, pickle, chutney and jelly known to civilization. I don't remember eating the stuff, but I do have visions of lying in bed, staring up at the top of the massive mahogany wardrobe that was filled with jars of rhubarb jam.

Before I began my new life in Tuscany, jam-making was not on my agenda. But there are plum, pear and fig trees on the property and the harvest is plentiful, so while the renovation was in full throttle, I thought I would have a crack at making jam. I got hooked—even though I had to cook on a camp stove. Making preserves is incredibly easy, and as you gain confidence, you can experiment with different combinations of fruits and with adding flavours such as ginger, chili pepper, basil, lemon and lime. The best part, though, is spending a happy, chatty afternoon working with a gang and then sharing the spoils of our labours. The little jars we fill capture the essence of summer, yes, but also the essence of friendship.

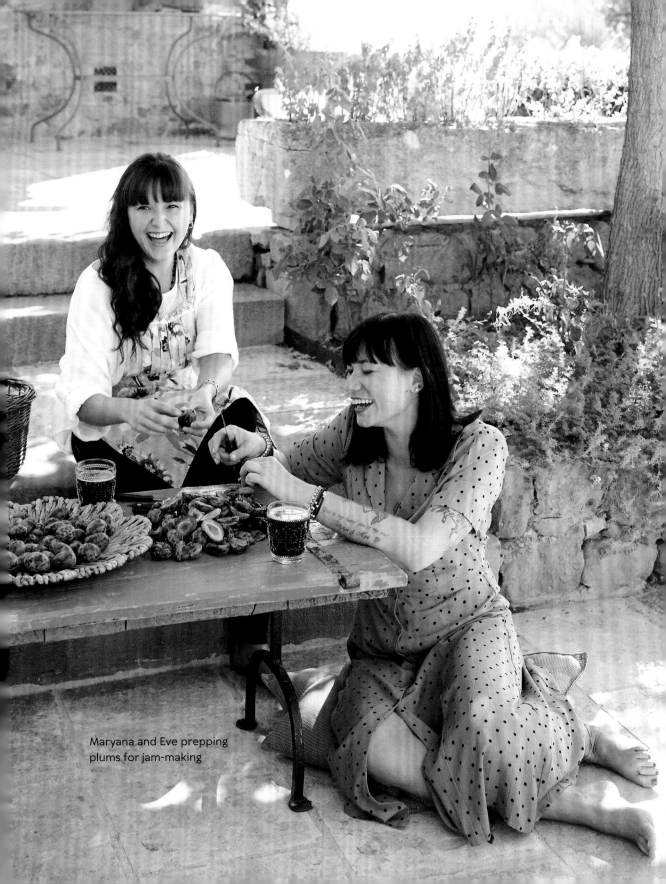

Maryana and Eve prepping plums for jam-making

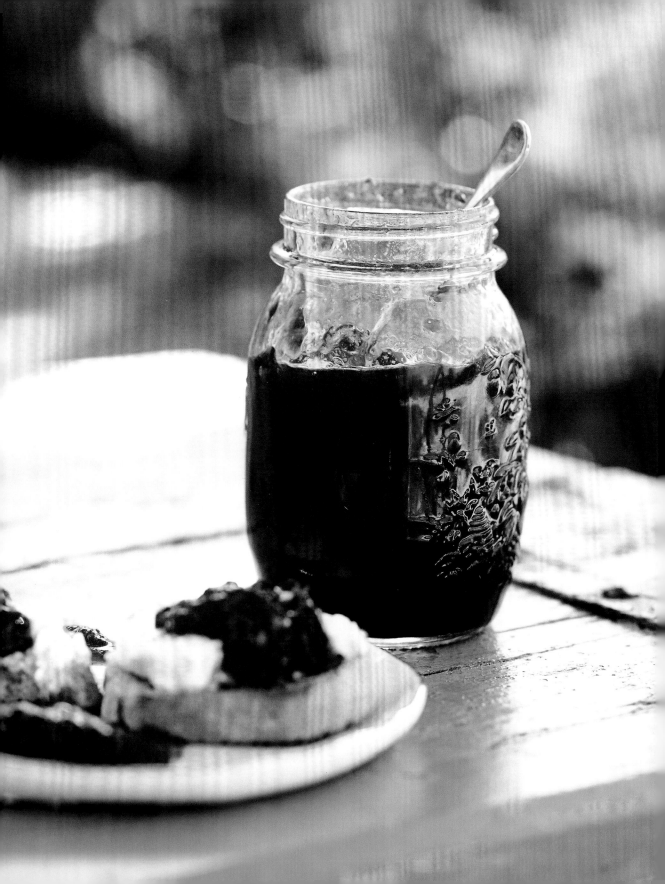

PLUM JAM

5 2-CUP (500-ML) MASON JARS OF JAM

I am new to jam-making, which I've discovered is not just for the experts—if I can make jam, anyone can. Actually, this recipe is more of a compote, because I only add a fraction of the amount of sugar you need for a traditional, long-lasting jam. You need to keep this one in the fridge and gobble it up within a month. I am using plums here, but you can apply this method to make the most of any fruit in season. I also love making jam with friends. A beautiful way to spend time together.

Choose plums that are slightly under-ripe as they make for a firmer jam than overripe ones, which are sweeter and softer. There is enough pectin in the skins of the plums to work without adding any extra. (In case you didn't know, pectin is the substance that sets the jam.) I love to eat this with chunks of aged cheese or on hot buttered toast.

3½ pounds (1½ kilos) plums, washed, halved
    and with the stones removed
2 cups granulated sugar
½ cup of whisky, rum or vermouth (optional)
1 teaspoon of cinnamon

Place the plums, sugar, cinnamon and (optional) alcohol into a large, heavy-bottomed pot, and bring to a boil, then turn down to simmer. As the plums release their juices, use a potato masher to smash the mixture into a lumpy pulp. I like to keep some of the plums chunky. Keep an eye on the jam, stirring frequently to make sure it doesn't burn, and cook for about an hour. As it cools skim off any foam that may appear at the top of the jam.

> **NOTE:** You can sterilize the jars and lids in the dishwasher. Or wash the jars and lids by hand in hot, soapy water and rinse (but don't dry!). Place the jars on a baking sheet in a preheated 325°F (160°C) oven for 10 minutes, and soak the washed lids in boiling water while the jars are in the oven. If the jars have rubber seals, boil these separately in a pot of water for about ten minutes, drain and lay on another clean tea towel to cool. Cover the lids and jar mouths with a clean tea towel, until you're ready to pour in the jam.

Take a Day Trip

I'm not talking about signing on for a day out with a busload of retirees here—though if you are a retiree, that's a wonderful idea. But what about recruiting a bunch of like-minded people to come on a day-long adventure with you?

The drive alone can be a recipe for hilarity. Hans and Steve are our retreats' designated drivers, happily ferrying our guests around to nearby towns and landmarks, and trying not to listen to the never-ending chatter from the back of the vans. "I am actually still here, ladies," they have been known to interject from the driver's seat as discussions of everything from uterine fibroids to orgasms to the horrors of liposuction ring in their ears.

Such trips can be a marvellous way to grow a small community of your own. Sally, who came to stay with us in 2019, realized on the retreat just what she was missing out on by living mostly for her job. After she returned home, she wrote me to say she was so inspired by the camaraderie on our day trips, she found a driver with a sixteen-seater van and approached the people in her yoga class to see if anyone was interested in sharing the cost of a day trip to the country, with lunch at a lakeside inn. Several jumped at the chance, and some brought friends along. The first expedition was such a success, Sally's day trips have become a regular thing, and each time the van is at full capacity. "It sounds silly," Sally says, "but this day trip sets me up for the workweek ahead."

Volunteer

An original Roman road—its large cobblestones worn smooth first by marching boots, then by centuries of horses, carts and local travellers—leads to what was once the main gate to our walled village of Montefollonico. Andrea, whom I'll tell you more about later in this chapter, is a much-loved community organizer around here, one of those people who just gets on with things. When he discovered that the road still existed, it was hidden under a carpet of ancient packed dirt. He was so excited by the

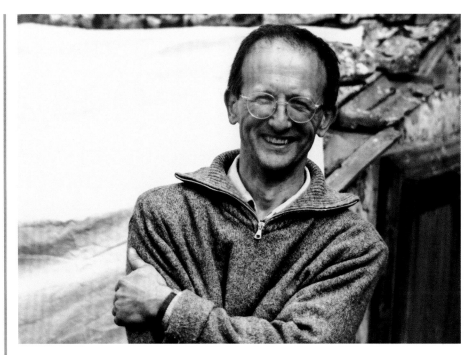

ANDREA

There is little point in owning a hillside property with a stunning view if it has no easy access to water—an issue we discovered after we signed on the dotted line. The solution? Andrea and his dowsing sticks. As the local specialist, he pointed us to where we could drill the exceptionally deep hole that produced a Niagara of water.

Dowsing is only one of Andrea's gifts. He is an extraordinarily kind soul who regularly brings people together for simple get-togethers and communal events in the village, making sure to include those who live alone. Andrea is the one who organizes a march in honour of the locals who died in both world wars. He runs the children's Easter egg scavenger hunt and, when the season rolls around, a family truffle hunt. All of us need a person like Andrea in our neighbourhood.

find, he began to excavate carefully around each stone with a dessert spoon. Soon, he'd recruited the entire village to come and help, bringing their own digging spoons, bottles of wine and panini. Even the tourists joined in. The excavated two-thousand-year-old road is now marvelled over by everyone who walks it, and the experience formed yet another bond among the villagers (and the helpful strangers).

Working together for a common good is an excellent way to build community ties. If you don't have an Andrea in your life, go online. In most places, you can simply google "where to volunteer" and a whole menu of opportunities will open up.

More Real, Less Virtual

We are social animals and we need interaction, friendships and people around us. But nowadays we've swapped a daunting amount of real time with others for virtual experiences. For many of us, it seems easier to post on social media than to pick up the phone, knock on a neighbour's door or go for a walk with a friend. And it's so easy to get dragged down the dark rabbit hole of endless swiping, filling the empty hours.

I know I just told you to search online to find places to volunteer, and I myself love to take a daily wander through Instagram and use such social media platforms as a way to share my ideas and passions. Even though I'm not hosting my own TV shows anymore, I still feel the impulse to communicate widely, and social media gives me the freedom to do just that.

But social media can cause us to forget our boundaries. While I share aspects of my life, I rarely mention my sons or my hubby, conscious that there has to be a separation between my real life and my social media presence. I think we can sometimes kid ourselves that we're the life and soul of the party because we have ten thousand followers, but this is a depressing fiction. A book club of eight people meeting once a week in person is worth more to your state of mind and your well-being than a million Facebook friends. A like or comment on social media—even from someone you know well—will never replace a warm hug and a proper conversation.

One Is the Loneliest Number

I know from talking with the many single women who come to the retreat (some widowed, some divorced and some never partnered) that the challenge of loneliness is real, and it can seem overwhelming to conquer. Humans are not designed to live a solitary life.

Yet I know myself that there is a big difference between being lonely and being alone. The first is to be avoided and the second is to be relished. At this stage in my life, having time alone feels like an absolute luxury, but I do worry about the future. There are so many ironies in the way we live. Because of social media, we are "better" connected than ever before, yet epidemic numbers of us suffer from a sense of isolation, recently aggravated by the lockdown in response to the coronavirus pandemic. Even writing these last few sentences has me welling up, fearful about the future, and running to the phone to call friends and check up on my kids, reminding them not to forget me when I am old! I am being melodramatic, I know, but who hasn't succumbed to scary thoughts about what our lives will be like in old age? But levels of forlornness are escalating in people of all ages, not just those approaching retirement—a trend accelerated by the coronavirus pandemic.

Also rising is the phenomenon of "weekend loneliness." My mother experienced a version of this when she was widowed in her midthirties. She was a beautiful, vivacious woman with many friends, and was invited to all kinds of get-togethers and events from Monday to Friday. But come the weekend, her married friends deserted her for their husbands at home. With four children to raise and boarders to feed, she was never exactly lonely, but I know she felt left out. These days, the weekend can be a sad wilderness for single working people. Some who live alone have told me that from Friday night to Monday morning, they rarely have a real conversation other than with someone in the supermarket. They dread the silence of the weekend, fearing their isolation will swallow them up.

Of course, we can feel just as lonely within a couple, and a single parent surrounded by kids can feel starved for adult companionship even while they can't find a moment for themselves.

There is a stigma attached to loneliness. It is a painful topic, one people often don't want to discuss for fear that, if they admit to being lonely, others will somehow view them as a failure. But actually, the biggest failure is *not* admitting that we suffer from social isolation, because that prevents us from reaching out to others and fostering new friendships. Believe me, there are plenty of people out there for

JACKY SAYS

The latest research on loneliness shows that social isolation is linked to physical and mental health problems from high blood pressure to heart disease to cognitive decline and depression. It is as if being alone too much acts like a bleak fertilizer on the body and mind, provoking diseases and weakening the immune system.

The English Longitudinal Study of Ageing (ELSA), is only one of the recent studies that confirm the health and social benefits of emotional well-being and connectedness. Its researchers found that, even if they have serious illnesses, people who live in tight communities where they have good support and regular social interaction are likely to live longer than people who don't. Feeling wanted and valued by others stimulates the release of the hormones oxytocin, dopamine and serotonin, which create that warm, fuzzy feeling of inclusion. The giddy feeling of a girls' night out—which we try to create every evening at our retreats with the *aperitivo*—is better than any drug!

you to connect with—you just have to find them. Try and then try again, because your health and well-being, and even your longevity, depend on it!

I sometimes look around my Tuscan village and wonder if the locals know just how blessed they are to live in such a close-knit community. One morning I was having coffee with a friend at the café, and she pointed to an elderly man sitting alone on the edge of the terrace. "How old do you think he is?" she asked me, and before I could answer, she blurted, "Ninety-eight!" The man was still handsome and had a full head of hair. I would have guessed he was thirty years younger than that. Inspired, we wandered over to ask him how he was, thinking he must surely know the secret to a vital life. We were crushed when he answered, "There is no illness quite as deathly as loneliness."

We returned to our coffees, heartbroken for him and the life's worth of friends and relations he must have lost to have inspired such an answer. But then we watched as over the course of the next half hour or so, he was approached at least a dozen times by members of the community stopping by to simply say hello. Then a great-grandchild perched alongside him for awhile and chatted away, followed by our barista. I could only think of how lucky he was to live surrounded by neighbours who care.

How to Bring Tuscany Home

- Stay positive by focusing on your good traits. This builds self-worth and in return makes you more interesting to others.

- Laugh with a buddy: humour can put life back into perspective.

- Find ways to bring your community together or create a new one. You can do it!

- Join or launch a community vegetable garden.

- Join a walking group, an art class, a baking workshop—whatever appeals!

- Take up a hobby. It's an amazing way to meet like-minded others.

- Volunteer!

- Reach out regularly to your friends and family. Relationships disappear when you don't take care of them.

- Contact people you want to stay in touch with, rather than waiting for them to reach out to you.

- Begin a conversation with a stranger at the hairdresser, gym, grocery store or garden centre. You never know where it will lead.

- Plan ahead for holidays and celebrations, to avoid being alone at these times.

- See your friends in person. Face-to-face encounters have the biggest positive impact.

- Be careful how much energy you spend on relationships that exist only on social media.

- Widen your circle of friends—include your friends' friends in gatherings.

- If you're lonely, know that you are not alone: banish the stigma!

- Embrace the spirit of the *aperitivo*. You don't have to serve the perfect meal in the perfect way to invite people over and have fun!

- Cook together! Many hands make light work of preserving jam or cooking a celebratory feast, and your friendships will be deepened too.

- Kindness is king. Keep an eye out for neighbours who live alone, especially the elderly. You'll work miracles just by finding an hour to sit and have a chat.

- If you have a spare room, think about renting it out to help a student or anyone on a tight budget.

- Understand that we are all fundamentally the same; simply being lonely does not make you a loser.

- If reading this list of suggestions and contemplating the changes you might need to make to widen your social circle feels really challenging, then seek professional help. You could be dealing with deeper underlying issues.

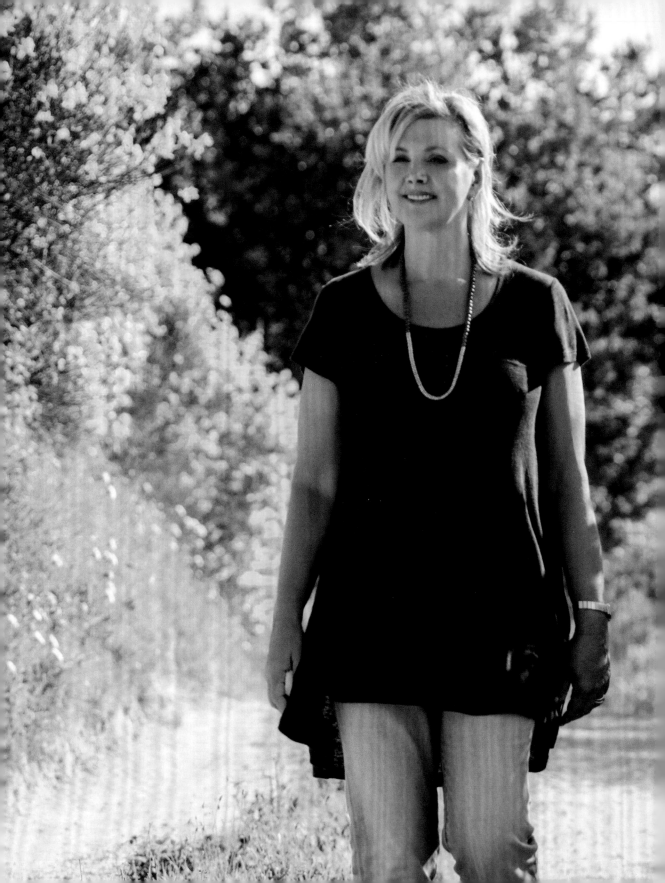

Live
with
Purpose

Open the Door
and Step Through

I AM CONVINCED THAT AN INHERENT SENSE OF PURPOSE lies behind the fact that Italians live long lives, with significantly better health, than many of us who live in other countries. An eleven-year-long study by *The Blue Zones* author Dan Buettner and his team looked at the relationship between feeling a sense of purpose in life and a healthy, vibrant old age. They found that people who play a significant role within their community—who feel needed by others—not only score higher on the happiness scale, but also live longer. They get out of bed in the morning because they feel useful, and like they matter to someone. In Italy, these attitudes are rooted in strong family relationships and traditions.

Some of us discover purpose through spirituality or religion, others through the art we make. Some are lucky enough to have a job that feels like a mission in life. At the end of the day, I think all of us find purpose through the relationships we cultivate. Rather than letting our roles—mother, lawyer, teacher, entrepreneur—define us, our true purpose depends on knowing who we really are as human beings. What is our authentic self, our unique character? What do we want for ourselves, not for others? Depending on how we define our value in the world, we can feel our secure sense of these things slipping away as we age. But that doesn't seem to happen as easily to the elders who live in the village and farms around our villa in Tuscany.

When we take guests to the weekly market, they always find the experience eye-popping—the bustling crowds, the stalls piled with produce, the bargains. But something else also startles them: "Why are there so many old people?" Instead of teenagers loitering and looking for trouble, Italian markets are full of gangs of retirees shooting the breeze, gesturing and poking and prodding each

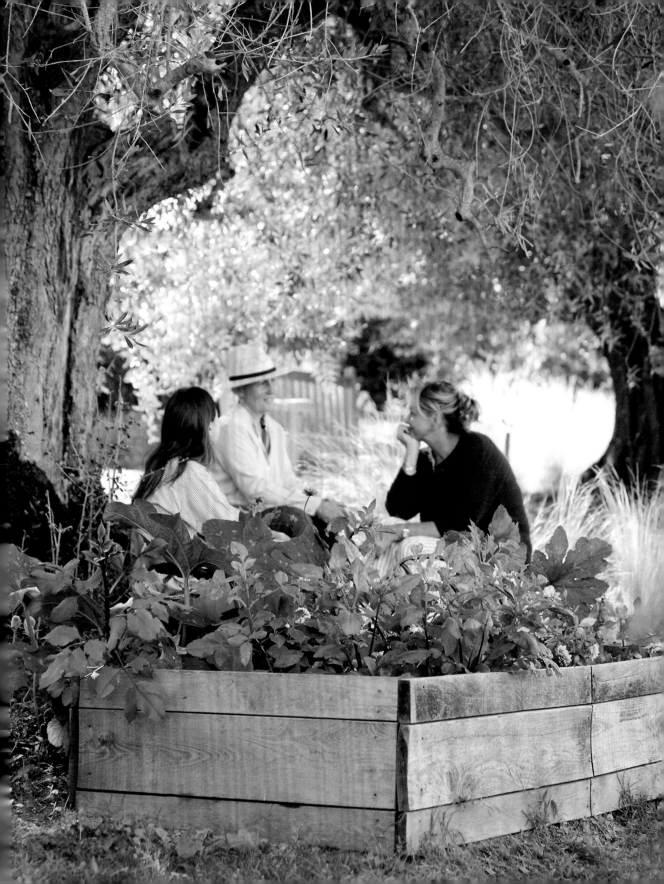

other with the familiarity of the schoolyard. Old geezers share tall tales while their wives shop, clutching a grandchild by the hand as they search for the best vegetables. The lines etched by time on these women's faces can make them seem stern, but occasionally they let out an absolutely girly giggle, often after they've received a compliment from one of the old guys, most of whom they've likely known since they were girls.

These lively and independent elders didn't wake up in the morning wondering what they were going to do with themselves. They have a role in the family hierarchy. They still have friends, and they have a context for their days in the almost unshakable local traditions. All of that together keeps them healthy, mobile and part of society. I think our guests find it surprising to see so many octogenarians in the market because of how old people have come to be regarded back home, segregated in retirement communities or living out their frailer days in long-term care.

After I did my first appearance on one of the home shopping networks out of Florida, I remember encountering a jewellery maker who was racking up colossal sales with her cheap and gaudy pieces. I must have looked surprised when she told me how well she was doing, because she immediately confided that her success was not about the jewellery but the delivery guy. "A majority of the television shoppers are lonely," she said, "and so when they buy something, which they do constantly, they get to open their front door to a friendly person bringing a 'gift,' which for a solitary moment makes them feel special. These people, for whatever reason, have little purpose in their lives." I can't tell you how saddened I was by her observation, but I couldn't dispute it.

Some of us are lucky enough to be born with a sense of passion that leads us through thick and thin. My elder son is one of those lucky ones, a humanitarian whose mission is to help others on a global scale. His compassion and skills take him to corners of the world where, for the thousands of refugees he works with, their purpose is simply survival—finding clean water, food and medicine. Their hope and aim: that their children will find a better life. I will never be able to compete with my son's big-hearted purpose, and I am lucky enough not to be a refugee, but I share something with both: the steady will to move forward. When stuck, I've always been able to find the passion to reinvent myself.

I feel such empathy when someone at our Tuscan retreats confides that they have lost their purpose. Often they sound as matter-of-fact as if they left it on a bench at the bus stop. *I lost it—where did it go?* Sometimes it was shocked right out of them. Life throws change at us, and not always for the better: the loss of a job we loved, the loss of a life partner through divorce or widowhood, the loss of our health through illness or accident. There are moments when all of us hit a roadblock or fall into a dreadful feeling of despair.

I will never forget Francesca, whose grandparents had emigrated from Tuscany to Texas. Recovering from a painful breakup, she decided to try to find her resolve by coming to one of our retreats. She ended up here on a particularly wild week when we were hosting five Australians, three South Africans, two Americans, one Belgian and six Canadians, former strangers who all got on like a house on fire (thankfully not mine). All except for Francesca, who spent most of her time sitting in the village piazza with the locals. I was worried about her, so one evening while the others were drinking their Aperol spritzes by the pool, I walked up to check on her. I found Francesca surrounded by a group of the village oldsters, who were telling her their tales of lives well-spent. When I asked her if she was okay, she responded with eyes shining. "Oh yes," she said. "I am discovering my roots. I am finding my purpose again."

So how do the rest of us find or renew our reason for being? You can't just buy a sense of purpose. There is no store you can walk into and say, "I'll have a kilo of purpose, please." Like everything else, finding your purpose is work.

The first step is as simple and as daunting as dumping the baggage we all carry around. If you aren't where you thought you'd be in life, stop blaming your background, the people who have damaged you and all the disappointments that have accumulated with the years. You don't need that stuff. It will just keep you stuck. Take the time to recognize your baggage and then set out to lighten the load by breaking the old patterns that block the way forward. Then, and only then, can you begin to discover what your life is meant for.

Learn to Value Yourself

When it comes to living a worthwhile life, there are no words more powerful than "love thyself." Well, maybe also "to thine own self be true." But being true to yourself starts with compassion, and it is never too late to befriend yourself.

A lack of self-esteem is often an issue for teenagers, and even twenty-somethings, but our sense of self-worth can also plummet as we get older, especially in parts of Europe and North America where the pace of life and the relentless youth culture can leave a person of middle age feeling like they have nothing left to offer to the world. This is something that is deeply wrong with our way of life, and it would do us all good if we could change it. In many countries, an individual's value *increases* the older they get. In Tuscany, the elderly are respected for the wisdom they bring to those around them after years of work and raising families, not treated as leftovers.

Whatever age we've reached, we must learn to value and love ourselves for who we are now, not who we were yesterday. There is no one, male or female, who hasn't looked in the mirror at some point and wondered, *Who is that person looking back at me? Where did those lines come from? When did I grow a second chin and, yikes, what is that suddenly sprouting from it?* Despite working as a model, I didn't shed my insecurity about my looks until I met Hans, who was nuts about everything that was me. Then my children were born, giving me an undeniable sense of purpose and unconditional love, and at last I grew comfortable enough with who I am that I was able to bloom, confidently painting the world and then creating television shows about how you, too, can make your world more beautiful.

So go back to the mirror and welcome the person you see there. Stop judging yourself! Be grateful for what you've been and what you've done, and for every wrinkle and wobble. The moment has come to find ways to value yourself for who you are now.

Give It Time

When life is a hamster wheel that never stops, we rarely have a moment to catch our breath and just be ourselves. It's easy to justify spending every waking minute fulfilling the roles people have given us: the beloved child, the fascinating lover, the perfect parent, the hard-working colleague, the good friend. But eventually a day will arrive when you ask yourself, *But what about me? Where am I headed?* And you might not know how to answer.

So take the time to do nothing but think. Keep a pen and paper close by. Seek out a quiet room or a park bench, and when thoughts come, which they will, jot them down. Try this for an hour once a day for a week.

The following week, put aside ten minutes a day to do something that brings you joy. Dance with abandon to your favourite song. Drink a glass of superb wine slowly, tasting the earth in which the grapes were grown. Learn something new, such as the history of the place where you were born. Visit the place where you were born. Sit in the park and talk to strangers (this is one of my younger son's favourite pastimes—he met the love of his life this way). Chase everyone else out of the house and prepare a meal of your favourite foods to savour alone. This isn't selfishness, but self-care.

Next, set aside a regular time to try something that takes you out of your comfort zone. Something you always wanted to do, but were scared to—even something you think you won't like. A couple of years ago I travelled on my own to northern India. Planning the trip was fun, but when I reached the airport to catch my flight to New Delhi, I was so terrified I nearly fled. It took every ounce of strength I had to board that plane, but I did and I'll never forget my epic adventure. The point is to shake yourself up. Here is where you start working on a new road map for your life. Again, keep it solo. Go climbing, learn to knit, learn to cook a completely new and foreign dish. The sky is the limit, but to figure out how to raise your enthusiasm for new ventures, you have to listen intensely to your gut.

Spending the day with yourself, getting to know the authentic you, is not an easy exercise. Remember that philosophers, pilgrims and spiritual leaders spend a lifetime searching for their purpose. Don't just say, *I'm too busy to take time for myself.*

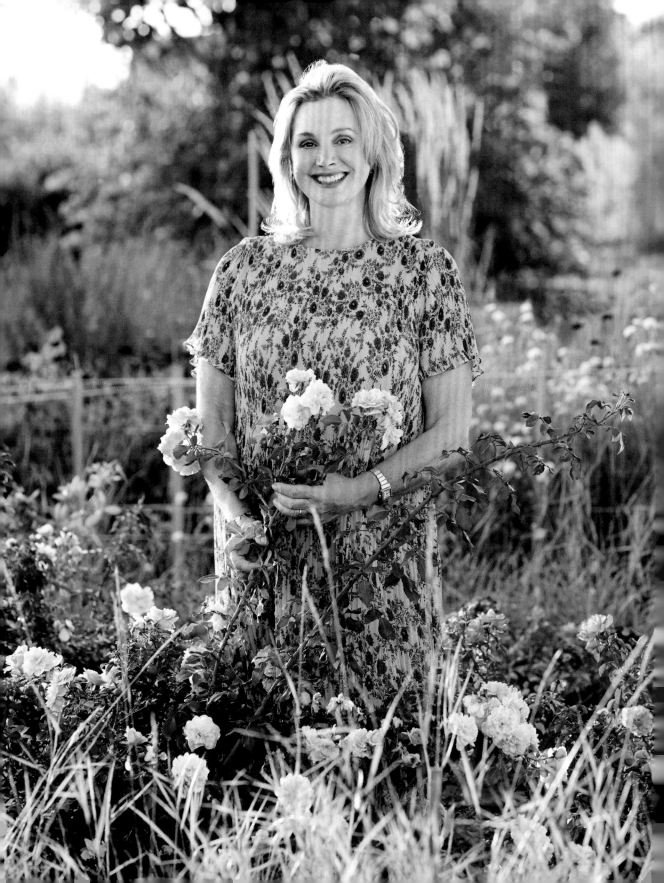

It's too easy an excuse in a world where people often complain about how busy they are. If you don't make time to spend with yourself, what is the alternative?

I cannot stress how well these simple exercises work. When I was halfway through the demanding renovation of the Villa Reniella, I had a panic attack. One morning, just as I had every other day for years by that point, I stood looking around at the piles of rubble, cement trucks and noisy bulldozers like oversized beasts gobbling up the earth. Hans was away, and I was on my own, directing the teams of builders, plumbers, electricians, plasterers and painters in a construction site the size of a city block. Suddenly I was so overwhelmed, I burst into tears, standing in the middle of it all, sobbing and shaking in my muddy boots. Eventually I realized I just had to get out of there. I went inside, wiped my tears and washed my face, took off my dirty jeans and sweatshirt and put on the prettiest dress I could find among my unpacked boxes. I am not sure what led me there, but I headed straight for a nearby flower farm. The Italian owners were all women, and extremely kind. When a stranger turned up out of the blue and asked if they could put her to work, they simply handed me a basket and a pair of garden shears. After giving me some basic instructions on the correct way to cut the many flowers they needed for the wedding they were working on, they left me alone. I spent the day lost in my own thoughts. I wandered up and down the rows of dahlias, daisies, roses and plants nameless to me but heavenly, staying until the sun had set. By then, after all those hours in my own company amongst the flowers, my doubts about whether I could carry the weight of the renovation had lifted and my sense of purpose was renewed.

When in Doubt, Ask Some Friends

Sometimes it's just really hard to bring who you are into focus. Once you have spent time alone, move on to others. Invite friends over for a meal or drink, telling them you want to pick their brains about what you could be aiming for. When the time feels right, give each person a piece of paper and ask them to write down what they think your gift to society is. Tell them to be honest—you can take it! Collect all the

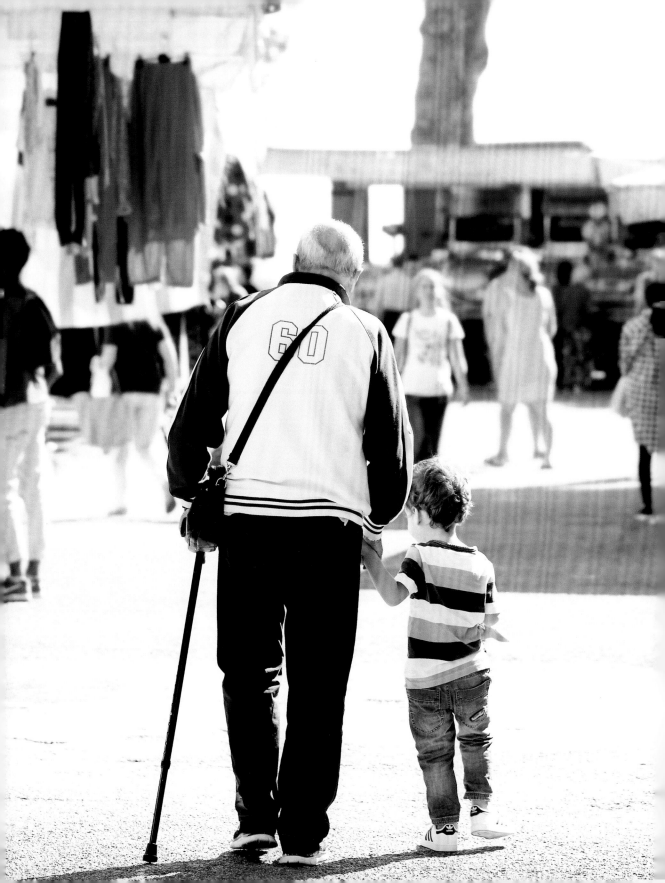

pages and then, after they've left, take a look at what they've written. Does anything stand out? Maybe they've described you as a good listener, a motivator, a great cook, a beautiful singer, a wiz with technology, an amazing dancer, a true friend, wonderful with kids. Is there a common thread? Even if there isn't, seeing yourself reflected in others' eyes can be illuminating.

Here at the retreat, our guests don't always know each other, so we do a version of this exercise where we each jot down a list of words to describe ourselves. When one woman sadly admitted that she couldn't think of anything to write, we told her to try again. She was alone after a tough divorce, with her kids grown and gone. She had a high-powered job in the tech world that kept her busy, but she had few friends. Eventually, looking gloomy, she read two words from her scrap of paper: *technically savvy*. The reaction from the rest of the women was unexpected. "Boy, do I need you!" "Come to my house and help me!" "What a talent!" The excitement went on for awhile, clearly astonishing her.

A month after the retreat, she wrote to tell me that she had thought about this exercise during her whole flight home, and she soon decided to put up a sign in her condo building lobby, offering her services for free to the people living there. She now holds one evening session a week in the common room, offering aid and support to her tech-baffled neighbours, who bring along wine and snacks and usually hang around for the whole session, chatting with each other and with her. She's made new friends *and* has found a purpose. She also met a man, but that is another story.

JACKY SAYS

Cultivating purpose leads to a fascinating string of benefits. A sense of fulfillment creates feelings of increased happiness, releasing dopamine, a neurotransmitter that plays a part in motivation, pleasure and learning, and other chemical messengers, such as serotonin and oxytocin, that are linked to emotional well-being. Clinical research reports that having a sense of purpose builds self-worth, and self-worth helps us gain the control we need to make better choices in life, including maintaining a healthy diet and regular exercise. All of these things are defences against depression and dark thoughts. A lack of purpose has the opposite effect, leading to boredom and isolation (and reaching for the cookie tin), all of which increase stress levels. Finding purpose helps us live a longer, healthier, happier life.

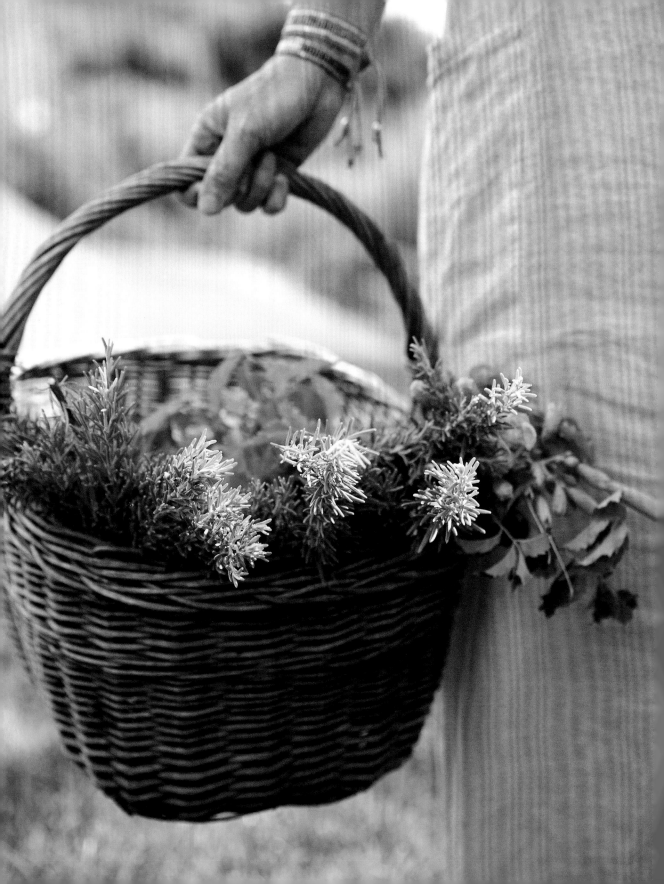

FRANCES

I befriended Frances Mayes when I first moved to Tuscany. The author of many books, including *Under the Tuscan Sun*, the iconic memoir that inspired me and so many others to dream of Italy, she finds herself still constantly captivated by the people here. I asked her what it was about their way of life that gave the Tuscans around us such a clear sense of purpose. She said, "Italians live in a time continuum that we adopted children can hardly understand. I'm from a tradition that values non-stop work. (How dreary!) But when I'm in Italy, I, too, step into this long time continuum where it seems natural to stay out until midnight on a random Wednesday night. To take the time to sit down in the piazza for a cappuccino with a friend. To take a spontaneous walk. Although the Italians I know work diligently, the job doesn't dominate their time or their thinking. Finding purpose can be as simple as making the most of the day ahead. My own writing life has been enhanced by the Italians' relaxed approach. And the work is more fun as well, rather than the North American nose-to-the-grindstone mentality. At the end of my week, I want to feel happy at what I've accomplished and to see a neat stack of fresh pages. This is my purpose."

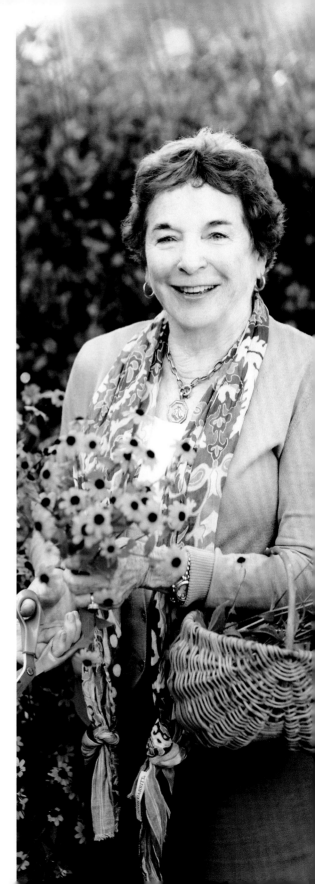

Let Yourself Be Curious

A curious person always has a purpose: to find out more about the world! Life is full of mysteries awaiting discovery, and curiosity is the engine that drives us to explore. Far from killing the cat, curiosity can ignite our lives. If you are curious about the world around you, you are, by definition, also open to new opportunities.

Jacky is the perfect example. She grew fascinated with investigating why a simple week in the Tuscan countryside, where women shared hikes, had cracking conversations and ate nutritious and delicious food without counting their carbs, had such a transformative effect on so many of them. What was going on? Back in London for the winter, she heard about a lecture by a renowned nutritionist and went to hear her talk on the subject of changing lives through the food people eat. She was hooked. Soon she'd found a school and made massive changes in her own life to allow her to spend the next four years studying to become a nutritionist.

We get so caught up in our endless busyness, we forget to be curious. We also sometimes think we shouldn't be curious, misconstruing it as nosiness. "Stop asking questions; this is none of your business!" I have heard that all my life, because I actually am nosy. I am fascinated by our world and by those who make it tick. I am interested in my Italian neighbours and want to know all about them, but I am just as drawn to the expats around us, who have acted on dreams similar to my own. I've been known to stop them in shops and restaurants and hit them with a barrage of questions. *What brought you to Tuscany? Did you give up your job back home, or are you trying to juggle? Did you put your kids in the local school?*

I'm not ashamed of my inquisitive nature. In fact, I revel in it, and I have met most of our new friends here by giving myself permission to ask them "nosy" questions. I come by it honestly. In the North of England, we like to know one another's business and we never hesitate to ask what's going on. If you're standing at a bus stop or are stuck waiting in a doctor's office in Northern England, I can guarantee that the person next to you will soon start grilling you on where you're from, what you do and even what you earn. I remember absolutely horrifying a woman who worked in television in New York by asking what her salary was.

Children have a natural purpose—to learn all the things they need to know to grow up. Curiosity is how they learn. To continue to grow, we adults also need to learn, to ask questions, to follow the trail of our inquiring minds at every opportunity.

My curiosity has helped me fit in with the locals. Just like my neighbours in the North of England, the Tuscans around me are fascinated by each other's stories—the good, the bad and the ugly. It is hard to feel like a stranger in a strange land here. The Italians are nurturing people, always with arms open, inviting you in for a glass of wine and a plate of pasta. Accept and you'll pay the price: they want to know all about you. Their curiosity is infectious.

How to Bring Tuscany Home

- Ask yourself what you want out of life.
- Don't be afraid to consult those you trust to help you see yourself and your talents more clearly.
- Reach out to people you admire and ask them what makes them tick, how they achieved the life they have, what pitfalls they faced and how they overcame them.
- Even if a major purpose in life eludes you, jot down a couple of intentions for the next year and check back on that note from time to time . . . you might surprise yourself.
- Grab every opportunity to learn. Be curious.
- Break out of your rut. Every week or so, try something that takes you completely out of your comfort zone.
- Engage with others. Support your friends and neighbours. Try to do a good deed for someone else every single day.
- Take one action a day, big or small, to help the environment.
- Take alone time. Don't think of it as selfish; it will help you get to know yourself.
- Tell that judgmental voice in your head to be quiet. Try your best to love and value all of you, inside and out, warts, wrinkles and wiggly bits.
- Use your talents to bring meaning into your own life and the lives of those around you.
- Understand that dreams change and so will your purpose. Change leads to personal growth, and personal growth keeps us vital.

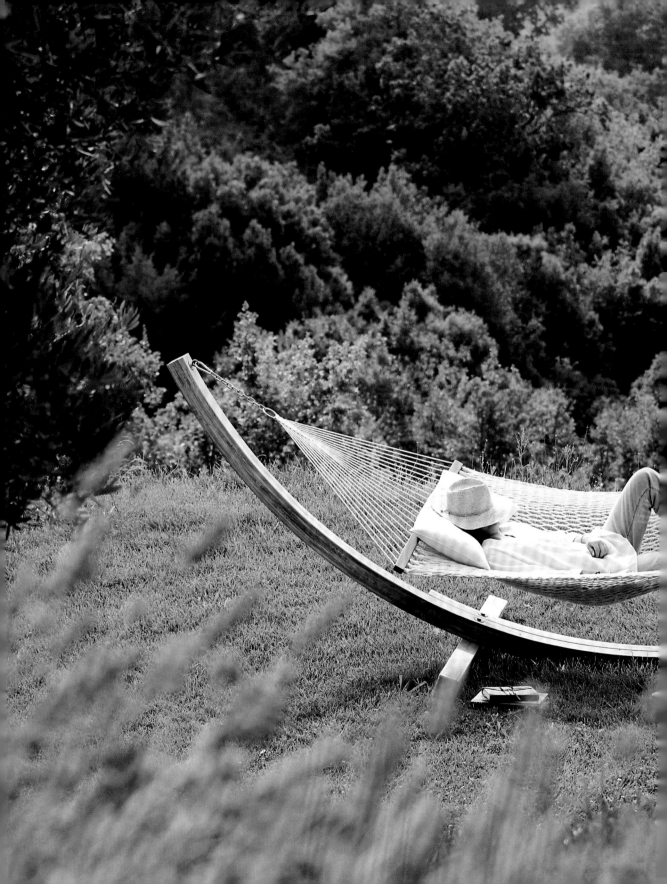

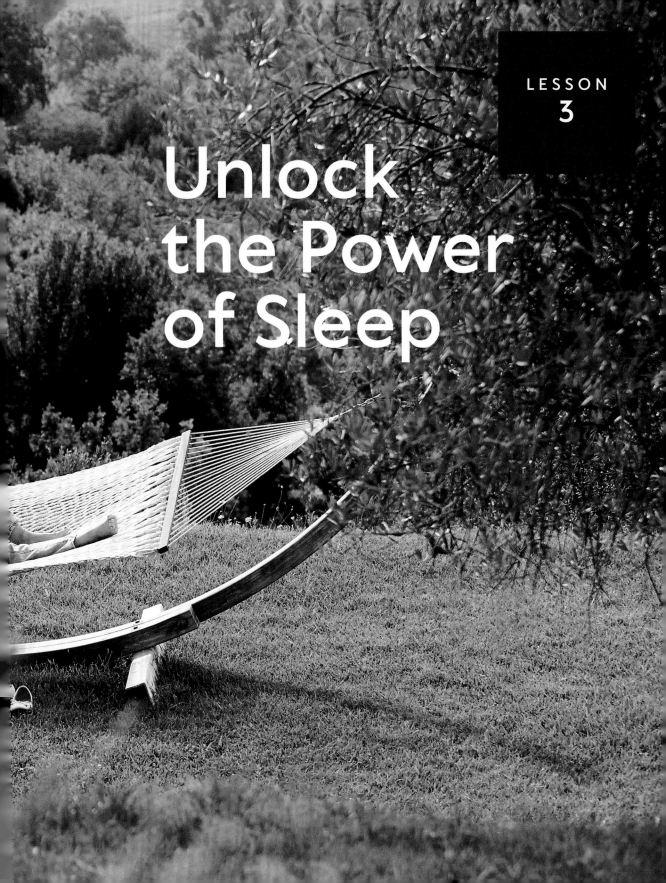

Unlock the Power of Sleep

Longing for a Good Night's Rest

YOU MAY BE THINKING you'll just skip over this lesson because you have no sleep issues; you are absolutely fine in the sleep department—you go to bed, scroll through Facebook for an hour and drop off easily. And what's the big deal, anyway? You've gone for years, functioning perfectly well, on very little shut-eye. But you would be wrong. If you are tired, it is impossible to lead a life oozing with vitality and full of joy. Exhaustion from lack of sleep spoils everything. It limits your capacity to be creative, limits the energy you can pour into your family life and makes it tough to meet the day-to-day challenges at work. Not to mention the stress caused by lack of sleep and the resulting impact on your health.

At the height of producing and hosting my television shows, I had a big problem with sleeping—I couldn't do it. I could *not* fall asleep. I tossed and turned all night, and by five in the morning, with my early wake-up call looming nastily, I would be so full of adrenaline I could have run a marathon.

I tried everything. I barred the kids from my bedroom in an effort to establish a place of calm and quiet. While I tried to fall asleep, I banished Hans to the sofa. I experimented with alcohol. When a few glasses of wine didn't work, I graduated to a tumbler of Scotch, which knocked me out but then caused me to bolt upright at two in the morning. I banned television, phone calls, electronic devices and work from the bedroom, yet sleep still evaded me.

One day, when I was waiting in the green room before appearing on a morning television show, I met an author who was there promoting a self-help book about sleep problems. I pounced on her with a barrage of tearful questions. I was desperate! Generously, she questioned me back, and soon she'd figured out that sleep was a problem for me only when I had an important workday ahead. On Friday nights, with no worries, I slept like a log. She explained that I likely couldn't sleep because my mind was too busy anticipating all of the challenges I'd face in the morning. Instead, she suggested, I should "panic about something trivial, something that will take place in the near future, like packing for a family holiday or figuring out what snacks to serve at one of the kid's birthday parties." (Carrot sticks had bombed.)

How would panicking about something else help me not worry about the next day? But whatever—I tried her suggestion and, while it took some practice, it eventually worked. Now, on the night before something challenging, I imagine lists of Christmas presents in my head, even if it's the height of summer, and gradually doze off.

Weirdly, as I think back on this stretch of being hyper-busy, it never occurred to me to ask my doctor for a prescription to help me sleep. Many of our guests show up for our week-long retreat with sleeping pills. Why have pills become the solution for so many? We all know that if we want to get into shape, we need to work out, or at least start walking every day; if we want to lose weight, we need to watch our diet. But faced with the way today's lifestyles wreak havoc on our sleep at night, we tend to either reach for the pill bottle or suck it up and suffer sleep deprivation. Some of our guests—even those who tell me they slept well—need five cups of coffee to get going in the morning. This has to mean they aren't getting anywhere near the rest they need. They're popping a pill to fall asleep and using caffeine to make it through the day, and worst of all, they think that's just the way things have to be.

We've got to change this way of thinking. Chronic sleep deprivation is a modern-day curse, but turning to medication should be a last resort. The American National Sleep Foundation recommends that all adults get between seven and nine hours of sleep a night. Think of those hours of rest as nourishment for the brain and a restorative for the body. Every night of sleep is like a fantastic spring cleaning. The night-long fast gives the digestive system a break, and the body is able to repair or shed damaged cells and remove toxins that have built up in the brain and tissues while we're awake.

I know I see the world in a whole new light when I wake up after a beautiful night's rest.

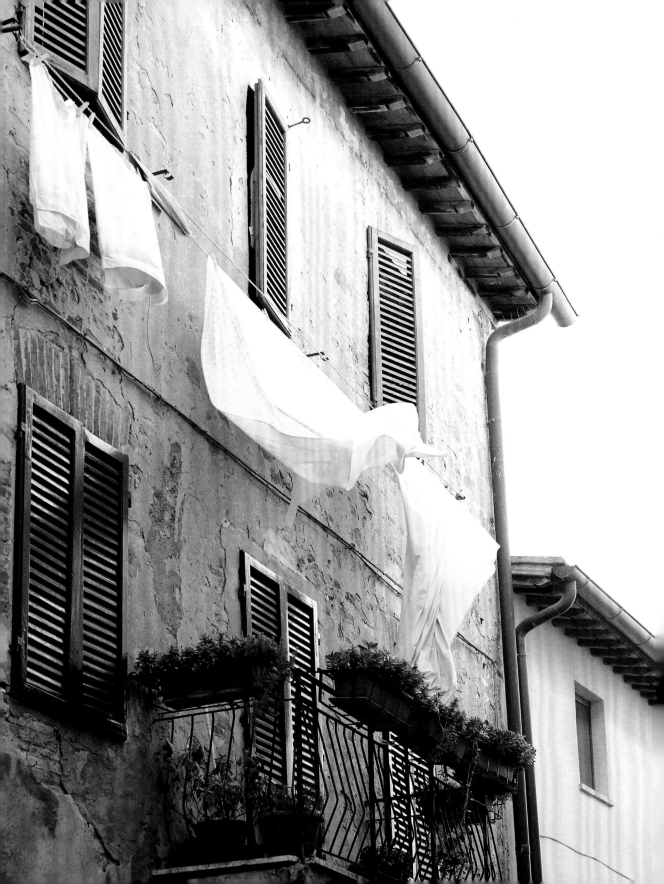

The Legendary Siesta

Walk the streets of any Italian town between one and four in the afternoon and you'll wonder where everyone went. Through a window partially open in the midday heat you might hear a typically animated conversation, but more likely the only sounds will be the wind through the trees, the rhythmic drone of the crickets and the occasional snore. Restaurants shut their doors around two, so if you want a late lunch, you are out of luck. Behind the closed shutters of the shops, the proprietors are taking a rest. Factories, banks and even police stations are usually closed until the middle of the afternoon as everyone practises the art of the pause.

I remember landing in Milan for the first time in my early twenties on a modelling assignment. When my employers told me that the shoot would stop for a three-hour lunch break, I was thrilled: here was my chance to shop! (Who doesn't want to shop in Milan?) Before I set off, I stopped for a quick cappuccino in a café, where I met a beautiful young Turkish woman who was about to do the exact same thing as me on her first trip to Italy. After we topped up our caffeine levels, we waved goodbye and set off in different directions, only to find ourselves, twenty minutes later, back at the same café—the only place still open. This time we ordered something a little stronger, and when the waiter came back with the *vino*, we asked him what was going on. Was it a national holiday? He laughed, then kindly told us that we had bumped up against the Italians' honoured routine of coming to a full stop at midday for a well-deserved rest. We had discovered the Italian siesta.

These days, I admit I watch with some amusement as North Americans, especially, wander the streets of our nearby towns, dumbfounded as to why all the shops are closed for hours at midday at the height of the tourist season. I can hear them thinking, *Why are these people sleeping when they could be making money?*

Actually, Italians don't spend the whole three-hour break sleeping. They spend it living. They cook and eat with their families, and they catch up on the news and what they've each been up to, and only then do they rest, taking a short nap that sets them up for the rest of the day. I am someone who always wants to be busy, yet I have come to accept and respect my neighbours' stubborn determination to take this time for themselves. A day interrupted by lunch and a nap still holds more than enough hours to make a living. And it turns out that a twenty- to thirty-minute nap recharges your energy and lowers your stress hormones. Why we people from hard-driving countries have forgotten this is a mystery. I remember asking my five-year-old what he enjoyed most about his first day at kindergarten and he replied, "Nap time." He was so right.

Thankfully, other countries are catching up to Italy when it comes to napping, even if they're not pausing everything for a three-hour reset in the middle of the day. Major cities are launching "napping lounges" with annual membership fees (so much more soothing than racing to the gym!) or thirty-minute rentals of a space to lay down your head. Massive international companies, such as Google, Samsung and even Ben & Jerry's, have decided that napping is not just for toddlers, and pride themselves on providing napping pods where employees can unplug and recharge. Most airlines advise their pilots to take naps during long-haul flights, and hospitals recommend that doctors working long shifts nap as a countermeasure to fatigue, which is so dangerous to their patients.

When I first landed in Tuscany—with an ancient farmhouse to renovate and a history of working 24/7 in the TV industry, where every minute costs money—a nap was the last thing on my agenda. I was also not a natural napper. But I soon took a leaf from the builders working on the property, who set down their tools at precisely one p.m., ate a picnic lunch and then curled up in the shade for thirty minutes' shut-eye. It turned out that when I added a noonish nap to my day, instead of hitting my usual three p.m. slump, I was able to carry on with renewed energy.

The Different Stages of Sleep

Sleep is a wonderfully complex process. Numerous reactions occur throughout the body as we prepare for sleep: over thirty hormones and chemicals are involved in getting us to doze off, keeping us asleep and waking us up. One of the most important is melatonin, a hormone and chemical messenger produced by the pineal gland

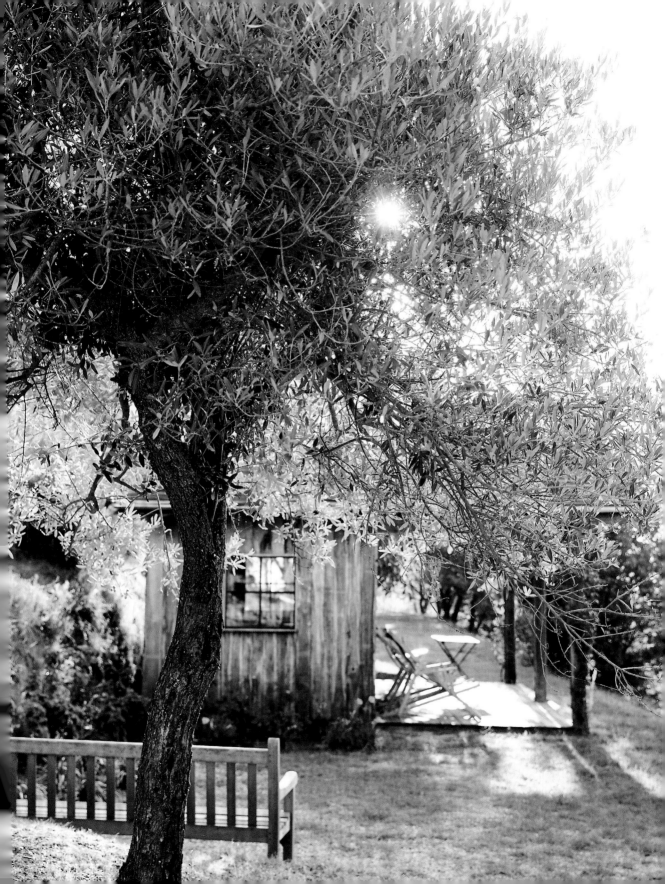

in the brain. Melatonin is stimulated by darkness. It signals our breathing and heart rates to slow down and our muscles to relax so we can drift off.

If falling asleep is your issue, melatonin supplements are available. People often find they work at first, providing some relief. Over the long term, the better, more effective option is to eat foods that contribute to the body's natural production of this hormone. Some foods that contain melatonin are cherries, walnuts, kiwis and bananas, while turkey contains an amino acid called tryptophan that the body needs to make melatonin (remember how sleepy you feel after eating Thanksgiving dinner?).

There are many nutrients that assist with sleep. One of Jacky's favourites is magnesium, a mineral known as "nature's relaxant." When our magnesium levels are low, we can fall asleep, but it's harder to stay asleep. Magnesium is found in leafy green vegetables, nuts, seeds, legumes, avocados and dark chocolate. It also comes as a supplement, and you can buy magnesium oils, sprays and creams for the body. For me, the most relaxing way to up my magnesium levels is simply to soak in a bath dosed with Epsom salts: the magnesium from the salts will help relax you and those tired muscles at the end of the day.

As we fall asleep, we drift into the first of three non-REM (rapid eye movement) stages of sleep, from which we can be easily aroused. After about ten minutes of this lightest of sleeps, we enter the second non-REM stage, in which our body temperature drops slightly and our heart rate slows further. We then move into stage three, or deep wave sleep. This is the crucial stretch during which the body repairs itself, releasing human growth hormone to restore muscles and strengthen the immune system. It is very hard to wake people who are in this third stage of non-REM sleep; it's the stage when they sleep-walk, experience night terrors and talk in their sleep.

About sixty to ninety minutes after we fall asleep, we reach the REM stage, when dreams happen. It's also the point in the sleep cycle when your brainwaves most resemble those of your waking brain; your eyes make rapid movements under your lids, but the rest of you is still and unmoving, and your muscles are sometimes paralyzed. (The theory behind that physiological response to REM sleep is that it keeps people from acting out their dreams.)

Each sleep cycle takes roughly 90 to 120 minutes, and the cycles repeat themselves throughout the night.

JACKY SAYS

The ideal time to take a short nap is after lunch, when the parasympathetic nervous system relaxes your body as it enters the rest and digest phase. For maximum benefit, keep your nap short. Sleeping for twenty to thirty minutes drops you into the lightest stage of sleep, from which you'll wake feeling refreshed and energized. Sleep any longer and you'll enter a deeper state that will leave you feeling groggy and fuzzy. If you nap later in the day, you risk disrupting your important night's rest.

Not only will naps boost your stamina to tackle the rest of your day, but chances are you'll be generally healthier. Scientists argue that there is a direct link between the practice of taking siestas in Mediterranean countries and those countries' lower rates of cardiovascular disease.

One more tip from Italy: if you drink an espresso right after lunch, as is the custom, you can take a twenty-minute nap before the caffeine kicks in and you'll wake up to a boost of energy. *Prego.*

Regular sleep deprivation, meaning sleeping less than six hours a night, slows down brain function, endangers your health and increases the chance of an early death by 12 percent, according to a study published by the Sleep Research Society, based on work done by researchers from Warwick University and the University of Naples. Lack of sleep impairs your emotional health, reduces creativity and stunts your ability to problem-solve. Unquestionably, it reduces your ability to do your job, and yet many careers seem to demand an around-the-clock commitment, leading many of us to wonder how we can both take time for a healthy night's sleep *and* succeed in our work life.

A deep sleep is as crucial for good health and optimal functioning as what we eat. Our body clock was set in place by natural cycles of light and dark, yet since the dawn of the electric age, we've been able to choose our bedtime, to our overall detriment. The relatively new phenomenon of blue light, which is given off by televisions, computers, tablets and cellphones, suppresses melatonin and stimulates alertness, shaking up our body rhythms even more.

And so we turn to medication. In the United States, the market for prescription sedative hypnotics and over-the-counter sleep aids is worth over $30 billion annually, and other countries are not far behind. Sleeping pills should be a last resort in dealing with insomnia. They may help you drop off to sleep and stay asleep, but their benefits are short-lived, and the drugs can be dangerous and addictive. Though there are several on the market that are said to be non-habit-forming, think how much better you would feel if you could find a natural path to the perfect slumber.

Stress and anxiety are the main culprits behind sleep deprivation. So let's try an exercise to help you figure out why you can't sleep. First, where are you in life? Are you in the super-busy stage where you're working all hours to establish a career or deep in the chaos of juggling work and raising kids? Are you dealing with a first baby? Are you menopausal, woken up by night sweats or that weird restlessness that sets in at two in the morning?

Enter your notes about your stage of life, and how it might be influencing your slumber, in a sleep journal. Then start writing down the details of each hectic day: how much time you spend staring at screens; what you eat and drink, and when; how you exercise and at what time of day. Note who you chatted with, even on the phone, and how much time you spent on social media. Think about whether these social encounters left you feeling invigorated and inspired or envious and depressed. Multiple studies, one of which was published in the *American Journal of Public Health* in February 2017, warn that the habit of scrolling through other people's lives on social media before bed is more likely to leave us agitated than peaceful. And you might notice that an evening check-in with a relative upsets you more than it calms you down.

Jot down exactly how much time you spend relaxing at the end of the day. Do you wind down by watching television, by having a comforting drink with a friend or by reading a book? What time do you turn off the last device at night?

Try this exercise for a month. I promise you patterns will emerge. Only when you understand what's robbing you of your night's rest will you be able to make changes that are more organic than reaching for a pill bottle.

Also think about the quality of your sleep, which is just as important as the length. Are your nights disrupted by noise, light, heat or cold, by the impact of heavy meals eaten too late in the day, by caffeine or alcohol? Does your body itself seem to fight sleep? Do you suffer from restless leg syndrome, sore hips that make it hard to get comfortable, indigestion, a frequent urge to pee, middle-of-the-night sugar rushes, worry, negative thoughts or even panic attacks? To change your sleep habits for the better, you must know the answers to all these questions so you know what you need to address.

In the remainder of this chapter, I make a number of suggestions that will help you improve your sleep. But don't try them all at once! Begin by incorporating just one or two of the tips into your bedtime routine. When you've adjusted, add another. In no time you'll find that you are reaping the benefits of your brand-new sleep habits. *Buona notte*.

A Bedtime Routine

The Italians around me here in Tuscany thrive on routine. By eight or so every morning, they tumble out of their local cafés, energized by their espressos and cappuccinos, and hop into vans, tractors, cars and scooters. Just try being on any highway in this country between eight and nine a.m. and you'll see what creatures of habit they are. Then, as I've already mentioned, at one o'clock, the whole world comes to a full stop to practise the religion of lunch and the art of the nap. Only *stranieri* (foreigners) would be rude enough to disturb a household at this time; the locals know these restful hours are sacrosanct.

The same goes for bedtime. If I were orbiting in outer space, I think I would see all the lights along the Italian boot go out each night at the exact same time. Tuscany is a region of farmers who wake with the sunrise to keep the strict deadlines that nature imposes on them, daily and seasonally. We can learn a thing or two from people who work the land about how a daily routine helps us live—and helps us sleep.

Routine is important because it boosts our circadian rhythm, the twenty-four-hour body clock that regulates our sleeping and waking cycles and controls our metabolism. If our sleep is constantly disrupted, we become fatigued and can put on weight. When we crawl through our days feeling tired, we tend to reach for caffeine and sugary foods that give us the boost of energy we crave, setting the stage for the onset of metabolic diseases such as type 2 diabetes. Even small alterations to our

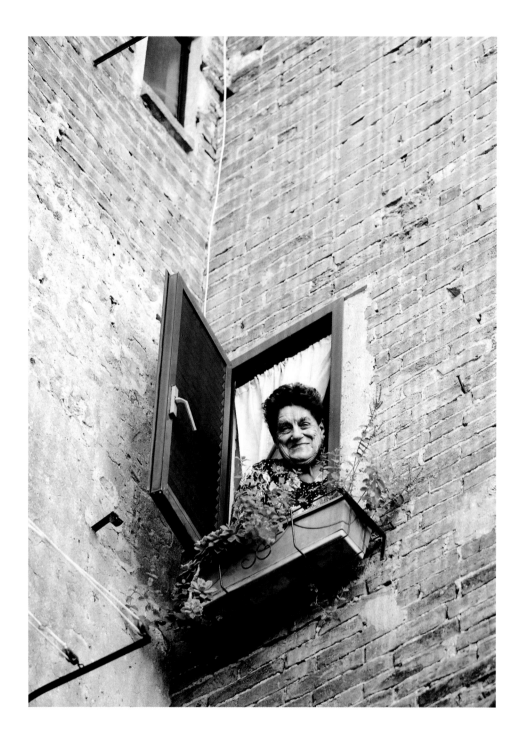

JOY

evenings—a slow-paced walk instead of an energetic workout at the end of the day, for instance—will reshape our circadian rhythm, awarding us the gift of a solid sleep.

Create a sleep schedule, and even if it takes time to kick in and deliver a night's rest, stick to it. Go to bed at the same hour each evening, and don't let yourself be tempted to finish that Netflix show. In fact, don't watch TV at all right before bed; you'll fall asleep more easily if you avoid bright light and blue light for a couple of hours before dozing off. Aim for a solid seven to nine hours, and keep to a regular wake-up time, too.

Of course, if you have young children, this may seem like an impossible dream, but a regular bedtime ritual for the entire family is a habit worth cultivating. And if you are in the throes of menopause, with night sweats and constant tossing and turning, battle through, just like you may have done when you had young children, and you will get to a better place. I promise.

Make It Cozy—and Dark

A dark room is crucial not only to help you fall asleep but to keep you in the Land of Nod. Any type of light can interfere with sleep. Light pollution in cities around the world has increased tenfold, and even a moonlit night, however splendid, can disturb our sleep.

This fact leads me to decorating, my favourite subject! Curtains are rare in an Italian home unless it's a palace or posh hotel. Instead, Italian windows are graced with two sets of shutters. I am now nuts about shutters and hung them on almost every window in our villa. Not just for their aesthetic appeal, either—they are a marvel of practicality. They moderate the heat of the summer day and keep out the winter cold, reducing energy bills. The slatted outside shutters provide ventilation, allowing air to circulate without having the window wide open, which is a huge benefit if you're attempting to sleep in the racket of Rome, for instance. The inside shutters are solid, and when firmly closed keep out all light, allowing for midday naps and a full eight hours at night in a completely darkened room. Did I mention I love shutters?

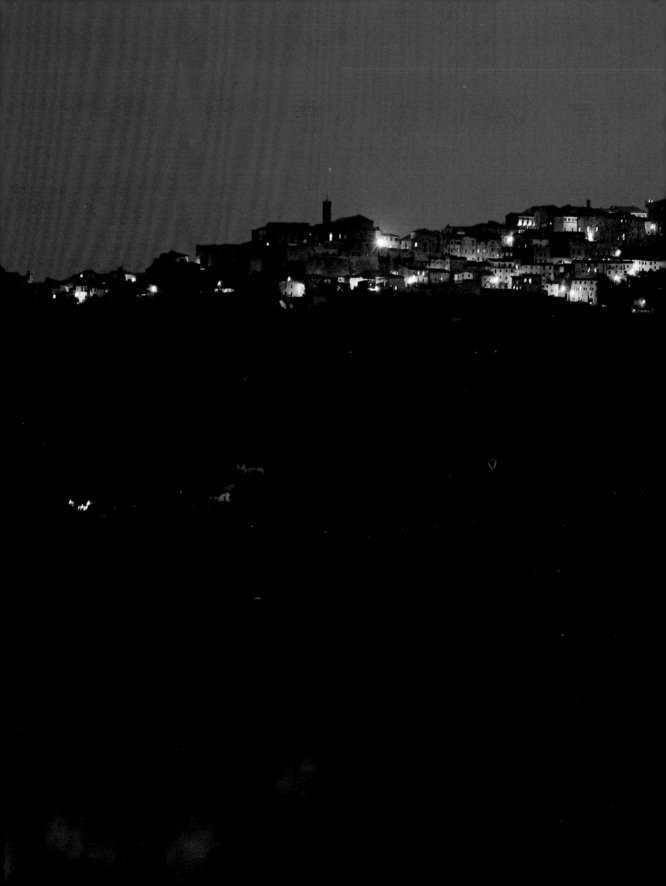

If you have blinds or curtains in your bedroom instead, ensure that they keep out the light. If they don't, have them lined or add blackout curtains. If that is not possible, wear an eye mask. (Jacky goes nowhere without hers. With her eye mask, ear plugs and special silk sleeping bag, she is quite a sight on a long-distance flight.)

And get rid of that digital bedside clock that both emits light and tells you exactly how long you've been staring at the ceiling. I have ripped a few out of hotel room walls (well, not really, but nearly) after lying awake watching the LED numbers ping through the hours. Unplug those clocks and invest in an old-fashioned alarm clock. It will wake you up on time, but it won't keep you awake all night. You may be tempted to use your phone as an alarm clock instead, especially when you're travelling, but that means keeping it on your bedside table, where it can be a constant temptation.

Turn Off the Blue Light

Take control of what goes on in the bedroom. When it comes to sleep, I mean. I was as guilty as everyone else of hauling my devices into the bedroom; there is nothing I like more than snuggling up in bed with my phone and my laptop on a chilly evening! But after learning how the blue light emitted by cellphones, laptops and all the other screens we tend to be addicted to messes with our internal clocks, I have stopped. It wasn't easy to break the habit, but not only do I now turn my devices off, I leave them outside the bedroom. Even better, I put them away at least two hours before I go to sleep. A sacrifice, I know, but the hubby gets more cuddle time. It is far too easy to give in to temptation and check Twitter or a news feed one last time at the end of the day, but if your cellphone is in another room, you will think twice. Then you won't just benefit from avoiding blue light, you might avoid a little late-night worry about the state of the world, too.

Shhhh!

If you live in the city, traffic, a neighbour playing music, a dog barking or people yelling outside your window can make it hard to fall asleep and stay asleep, given that the brain continues to register sounds. Oh, and don't be fooled about the "peaceful" countryside: it can be just as noisy. My neighbouring farmer loves nothing more than plowing his field at sun-up, and those chickens of his will be the death of me. If, like me, you prefer to sleep with the window open, ear plugs may be the answer. Or there are white noise machines that supply soft, steady sounds, such as rain or waves crashing on the shore, that can rock you to sleep, masking disruptive noises. Though I've recommended leaving your phone outside the bedroom, you can download apps that issue white noise, relax you with guided meditation or tell you bedtime stories. If one of these apps works best for you, set your phone to night mode to reduce the blue light.

Keep It Cool

For optimal comfort, keep the temperature in the bedroom cooler than the rest of the house: lowering your body temperature will help you sleep. Aim for a room temperature between 17°C (65°F) and 21°C (71°F). I can hear some of you muttering about night sweats; keeping the room cooler will help you, too. Keep a fan handy. You can turn it on when you're boiling and off when you're back to normal. Children and older people may need their bedroom to be a little warmer. It's an expense, I know, but it really is worth fitting each bedroom with its own thermostat so the occupant can set it to the temperature that suits them best.

Create a Comfy Refuge

Decorating shows, of which I've made my share, usually describe the kitchen as the soul of the house, but I believe it's the bedroom. It is where we start and end each day, and how well we sleep in it dictates how a day will unfold. The bedroom should be a calm and peaceful sanctuary.

When I designed the suites at Villa Reniella, my goal was to make each guest feel totally embraced by comfort and beauty as they settled in for an epic night's sleep. I kept the rooms simple and uncluttered. The walls are a whitewashed plaster. There are a few colours I avoid in the bedroom: reds and oranges are stimulating, so are not the best choice for a perfect night's sleep; yellow can feel aggressive unless it is an earthy or buttery tone. (I also avoid greens, as they tend to make me look sickly, and I prefer as much help in the bedroom as possible.) Try off-whites, pale greys, creamy tints, delicate pinks or pale blues. In my Tuscan guest rooms, I added a splash of colour and personality by tucking vibrant lime and pink throws over the alabaster linens and installing patterned headboards.

The most daunting task was purchasing the mattresses for the villa. I needed more than twenty, and they had to work for every possible body type. Choosing a mattress is so personal—how could I possibly get it right for each individual who stayed with us? Then I slept overnight at a nearby bed and breakfast and woke up with my weary bones fabulously rested. Oh, what a sleep! The mattress was perfect: not too soft, not too hard, and made from hypoallergenic sheep's wool. My hosts told me the manufacturer, and I immediately got in touch and purchased enough for the entire villa. I am reminded how fabulous they are each morning when guests wander into the kitchen boasting about their idyllic sleep.

Quality mattresses can be wildly expensive, I know, and even the best of them should be replaced every eight to ten years. If yours is sagging and uncomfortable, it is time to bite the bullet or risk not only losing sleep but waking up stiff and sore. Always test mattresses out in person, and remember that if they are either too hard or too soft, they can cause hip, shoulder, neck and back problems.

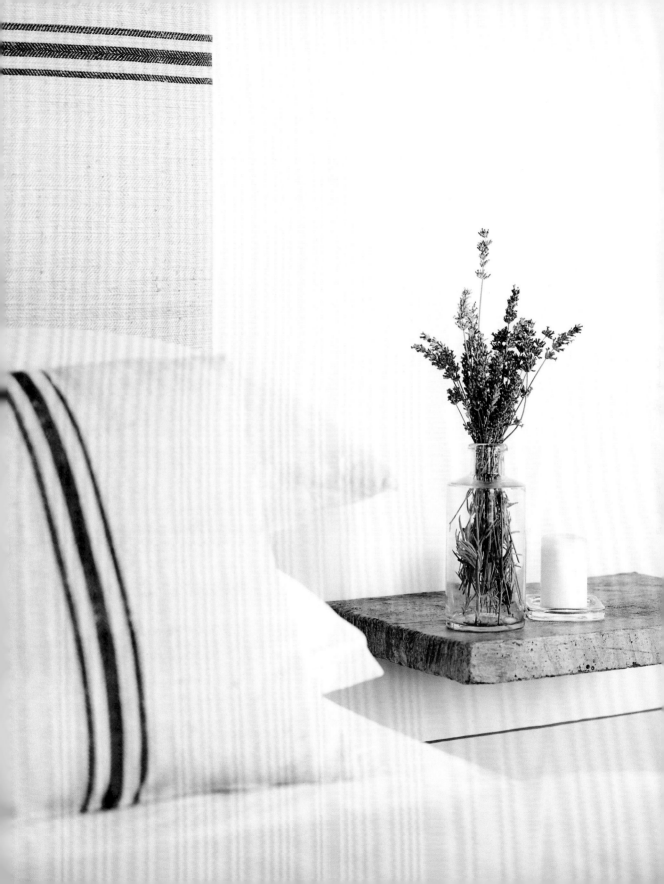

Once you've found the mattress that suits you best, choose the best linens you can afford. There is nothing quite as luxurious as crawling into a freshly made, heavenly comfortable bed. You might prefer crisp hotel-style sheets, but there is a growing trend for rougher Italian linen that breathes beautifully in the summer months.

Pillows are like mattresses, with a buffet of stuffings: feather, down, memory foam, microbead, buckwheat—even water-filled. Choose the one that suits you best, and remember to use a pillow cover, which will prolong your pillow's life. Most pillows need to be replaced about every two years.

You will need to rest after all this testing, but it will be worth it.

Perfumed Nights

I became intrigued by the benefits of lavender after a visit to a lavender farm in the South of France. After we bought our own place in Tuscany, I decided to plant a field of this robust herb because the summer temperatures are similar here to those in the South of France, and so is the stony, dry soil. My lavender now grows with the ferocity of a weed. I harvest it every year, and use it to create a variety of products. I rarely travel without a tiny bottle of organic essential oil made from my own plants. Studies have found that a couple of drops of lavender oil on a pillow, on a sleep mask or in a diffuser decreases your heart rate, lowers your blood pressure, eases restlessness and helps you drop off. Even a lavender plant kept on your bedside table will exude soothing scents that help induce sleep.

Our response to scent is deeply personal, though, and there are many other plants with calming effects. Ancient Romans fell asleep to the relaxing scent of chamomile, and the ancient Egyptians burned cinnamon. The comforting aroma of vanilla makes us feel more positive; sandalwood, juniper and bergamot are all stress relievers; marjoram has a calming effect, helping us relax; and lemon is uplifting and improves our mood. Try adding a few drops of essential oil from any of these plants to a diffuser for a restful sleep.

MR. TROMBETTI

An elderly man, squat and solid, greeted me with his familiar broad grin as I joined him in the bar for a beer. Marcello Trombetti lives within the stone walls of the village now, but he spent his childhood and working life as a farmer at what is now my home. He's always friendly. I love his stories about the old days, and soon I was grilling him for tips on living a full and vital life. He was a little reticent when it came to such tips until I mentioned how happy he always seems and how handsome he is (there is no one quite as vain as an Italian man). Then he opened up and told me that the life of a farmer is about routine. "I wake with the cockerels and close my eyes when my wife tells me to," he said, and roared with laughter.

"But tell me, why are you always so full of joy?"

"Well," he said, "*dormo bene* [I sleep well], with no worries because I live in a neat, small apartment in the centre of the village, and I am comfortable now because of all the money from the old ruin of the farm I sold. I'm as happy as the pigs who lived in what is now your living room. Why would I not smile all day?"

It was not quite the answer I expected, but it made me laugh. As I walked away, he shouted after me, "*E niente latte prima di coricarsi!*" ("And no milk at bedtime!")

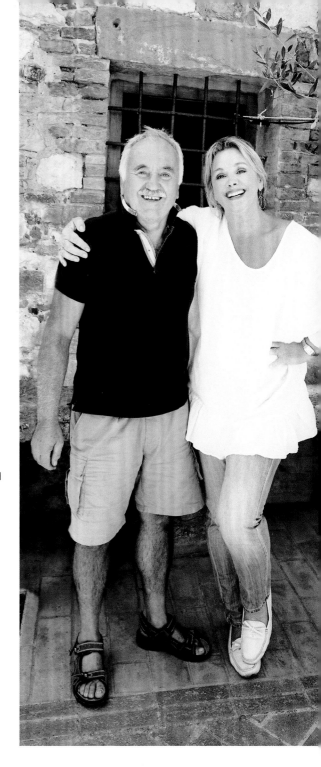

Watch What You Eat and Drink Before Bed

Italians tend to have dinner later than North Americans usually do, but they eat a light meal—unless they're celebrating, and then it's a feast! In Italy, lunch is the most substantial meal of the day, which makes good sense when it comes to digestion. The digestive system functions better when we eat during a twelve-hour daily window, allowing the gut to rest and repair itself during the night. But for many of us, maintaining a regular, sensible mealtime is challenging. If you must eat late in the evening, choose easily digestible foods rather than big hunks of meat, deep-fried foods or mounds of raw vegetables (save those for the daytime). The best options for late-night sustenance are soups, broths, scrambled eggs, sweet potatoes and cheesecake. (Kidding about that last one.)

Remember your granny telling you that eating a cheesy snack before bed would give you nightmares? She was right. Cheese takes a long time to digest, so if you prefer sweet dreams, eat cheese earlier in the day. And try hard not to munch too close to lights out. Think of all the work a heavy meal asks your poor body to do after a long day. Just the thought of a burger and fries before bed has me propped up against a pillow burping.

Then there's our caffeine habit. Caffeine is a powerful stimulant that activates the nervous system and sets our muscles humming. It takes five to six hours for caffeine to leave the system, and even longer for some of us. That coffee you grabbed after lunch may still be racing around your body at bedtime; when you take in too much caffeine, it's hard for the liver to metabolize, and as a result, it builds up. Jacky says caffeine really affects adenosine, a sleep support hormone (along with melatonin and others). Our adenosine levels rise towards bedtime to initiate sleep and keep us asleep. During the night, adenosine levels slowly decrease, allowing us to wake up alert and refreshed. Caffeine blocks the receptors for adenosine, which is why a cup of coffee too late in the day may make it hard to fall asleep. If you're plagued with insomnia, try avoiding coffee, tea and sugary drinks that contain caffeine altogether for a few weeks and see how it affects you. You may witness a wee miracle.

And don't be fooled by the sedative properties of alcohol. I mentioned my own experience with trying to knock myself out at night with a glass of Scotch. I have also watched my hubby doze off many a time after a nightcap of whisky. But like me, he always wakes up two or three hours later. Alcohol is incredibly disruptive to sleep patterns. A delicious bottle of wine drunk with dinner may seem a delightful way to be rocked to sleep, but several hours later the sugar rush from that robust *vino* will have you wide awake, depressed and vowing "never again." Try taking a break from booze for several days a week—even for a solid month. It can be a game changer.

I love nothing more than an evening out, eating and drinking wine, but I've learned I will suffer afterwards. Now I regularly abstain for weeks or even a month. I actually look forward to these times now: I feel so good and sleep so well, waking up ready for the new day. (But I still love a glass or two of wine, I have to admit.)

Deep Breathing, Gentle Yoga and a Warm Bath

If falling asleep is an issue for you, research shows that slowing down your breathing and taking deep breaths stimulates the parasympathetic nervous system and assists in quieting the mind, reducing anxiety. By practicing slow, deep breathing mindfully after we climb into bed, we can soothe ourselves to sleep. A gentle yoga session or meditating before bed can also lead to a calm state. Follow this up with a warm bath, and you will be out like a light.

Sex Is a Funny Thing

Even though desire definitely wakes us up, a good old tumble actually helps us fall asleep. Better yet, getting a good night's rest boosts your sex drive.

I know: at some stages in your life, especially after a day spent working flat-out at a job and then chasing kids, sex can be the last thing on your mind. But sex sparks the release of some important hormones, especially oxytocin (the cuddle hormone), that cause us to feel serene and happy, and it lowers cortisol (the stress hormone).

Jacky says that, by regulating the body's blood sugar levels and metabolism, cortisol helps keep us vital, motivated and awake during the day. But too much cortisol on a regular basis causes problems. Cortisol levels should peak in the morning, when we are active, and not at night as we lie in bed. But in a really vicious circle, lack of sleep stresses us, prompting the brain to call for a steady stream of cortisol, which stimulates continuous glucose production and inhibits insulin, the key to cellular absorption of glucose. If glucose is not used for energy, the body stores it as fat, contributing not only to weight gain but to depression, anxiety, insomnia and heart disease.

The dreaded deed, as I like to call it, is a lovely way to break this vicious circle. Orgasms also release prolactin, which relaxes the body and puts us into a drowsy state. Getting enough rest is the best way to counteract the stress hormone.

Sex has an added bonus for women: it increases estrogen levels, which heighten our REM sleep.

A nighttime cuddle is a very good thing.

How to Bring Tuscany Home

- Keep a sleep diary.
- Create a sleep routine.
- No television, laptops, social media two hours before bedtime.
- Remove all devices from the bedroom before lights out.
- Design a dark and tranquil bedroom.
- No heavy meals or too much alcohol for the two to three hours before bed.
- Work out earlier in the day and do only gentle exercises in the evening.
- Set aside ten quiet minutes for meditation or yoga before turning in.
- Make time for a cuddle: sex helps us sleep.
- Or take a hot bath to relax.

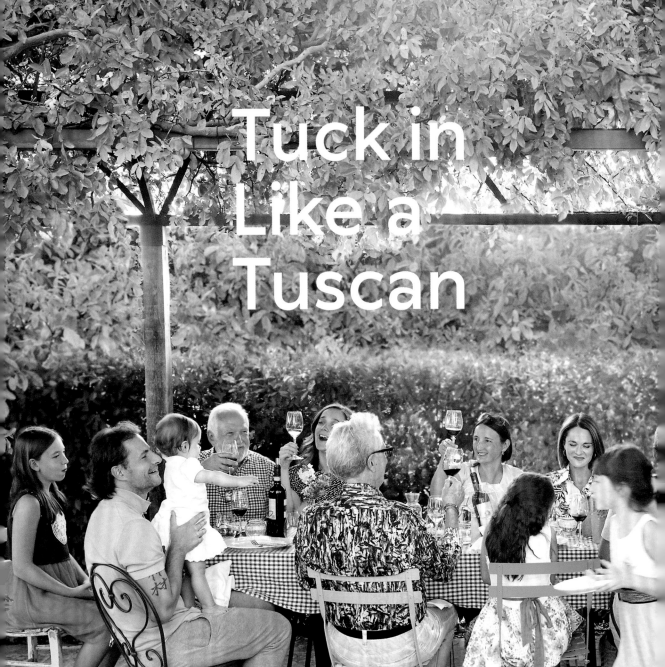

Tuck in Like a Tuscan

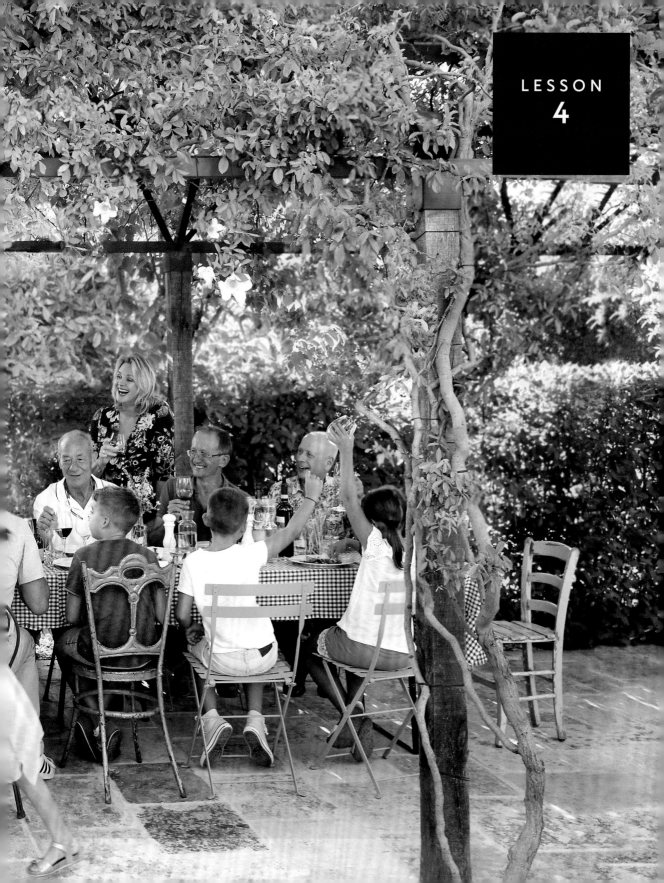

The Wisdom of the Italian Meal

YOU CANNOT WRITE A BOOK THAT EMBODIES THE JOY and vitality of Italy without talking about food and eating together. Rich, exhilarating and welcoming, Italian meals are the heartbeat of this country. If I could capture Italy's essence in a jar, I would unscrew the lid on a gloomy day to let out the glorious sunshine. I would release the delicious aromas of the Italian kitchen and the cheerful sounds of families cooking together, preparing and enjoying humble meals that are all about simplicity and goodness.

Italian cuisine allows fresh, local ingredients to be the main attraction, rooted in tradition and the diversity of the numerous regions. In centuries past, the boot-like peninsula consisted of hundreds of different states and principalities, each with their own governments, cultures, currencies and cooking methods. In the mid-1800s the Republic of Italy was created, uniting most of the regions. Still, practices, attitudes and food remained distinct, nowhere more so than in Tuscany, where gastronomic disputes rage on. Arguments over which village cooks the best tomato sauce have caused many a war!

Tuscany's contrasting landscapes include a long-reaching coastline, rugged mountains, endless plains and bucolic rolling hills. Hundreds of towns, villages and tiny ancient enclaves dot the land, and, of course, there are the glorious Renaissance cities of Florence and Siena. Geography and history dictate how the population eats, even today. For example, Villa Reniella lies in the east of the region, a ninety-minute drive from the sea. But in the times of the horse and cart, it was a full day's expedition,

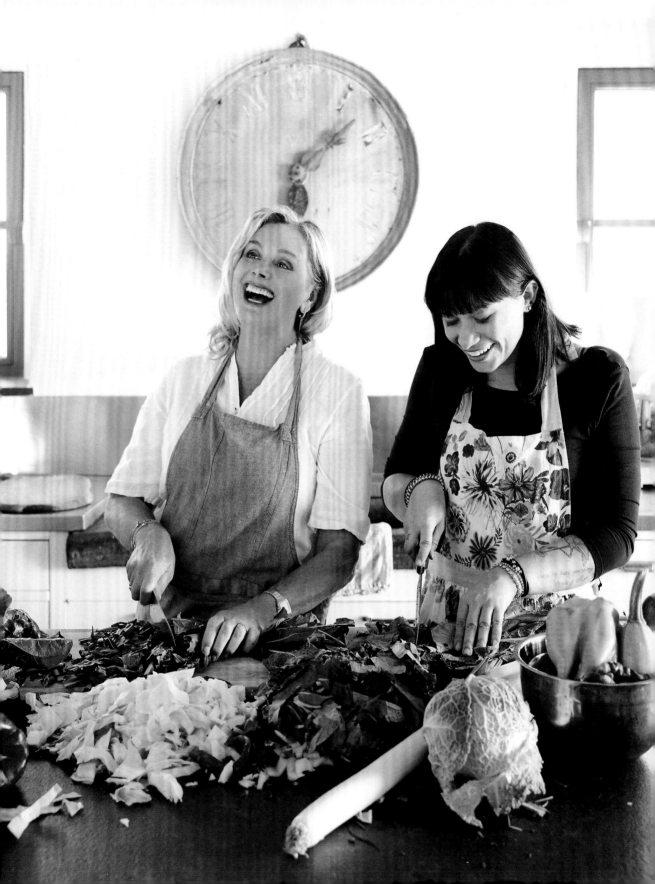

too long a journey for the unrefrigerated bounty of the Mediterranean to remain unspoiled. To this day, "inland" Tuscans, as true traditionalists, consume fish only on special occasions.

The Mediterranean diet is the norm throughout Italy, France, Spain, Portugal, Lebanon, Greece, Turkey and North Africa, all regions that share the same fundamental ingredients. For centuries, these peoples' nourishment has come from foods harvested locally: extra virgin olive oil, beans, grains, an abundance of fresh seasonal vegetables and copious varieties of herbs. Fish and meat are consumed in small amounts. The Mediterranean diet is now well documented as being balanced, highly nutritious and a leading factor in greater longevity.

After a week of savouring Tuscan food, our guests always comment on the wonder of relaxed meals brimming with chatter, mouth-watering delights and plenty of *vino*. As the week draws to a close, the inevitable questions arise: "Have I put on weight after three Italian meals a day?" and "How can I bring this way of eating home with me so I can hold on to this sense of well-being?" The answers are a delicious surprise. Most guests actually drop a few pounds during their stay and feel invigorated and healthy. As for bringing it all home, allow me to take you on a food journey that is accessible wherever you live. The only requirement is an open mind and a willingness to put all these life-changing elements into place. Let's tuck in.

When Food Is a Lifestyle

We are social creatures and throughout history the sharing of food has become synonymous with friendship, love and celebration. There is a deeper purpose to gathering people together, and I always want to find room for more guests at the table.

The first dinner party we held in the newly renovated villa was an eye-opener—it was our introduction to the drama that inevitably unfolds at Tuscan events. We had invited a mix of twenty-five new friends, both expats and locals. We had a long, beautifully decorated table set up under a pergola covered with climbing roses, and when our guests arrived, they sat down to large platters of *antipasti*. Francesco, the chef who cooks at our retreats, had offered to help with the meal. I was chopping vegetables with him in the kitchen when Hans burst in and asked who on earth all these people were.

Stepping outside, I saw that the dinner crowd had swelled to about forty. More strangers were coming down the driveway, clutching bottles of homemade wine and a variety of freshly baked sweet pies. Some of our friends were grabbing garden tables and benches and casually passing them over the heads of guests to extend the seating. Our architect had brought along his elderly mother, who wanted to see what had been done with the old place. Guests had brought guests of their own, and a small children's table had been erected in a corner of the garden. Surveying the bustling scene, Hans was quietly pulling his hair out.

Back in the kitchen, I whined a desperate "What the @*&$!" to Francesco, who remained the picture of calm. "*Normale!*" he shouted to me over the head of someone I'd never met who was busy taking over the kitchen. "We'll just put on more pasta. Relax, Debbie!"

Five years and countless gatherings later, the shock of no one calling beforehand to ask if it would be convenient to bring their neighbour or long-lost cousin has disappeared for good. It has become completely *normale*. I've embraced the Tuscans' unashamedly celebratory way of life, where any excuse will do to gather a crowd, throw some tables together and boil some pasta.

There is no greater joy than eating with friends, so go ahead—don't wait for a particular occasion; grab the phone and get a gang over to your place.

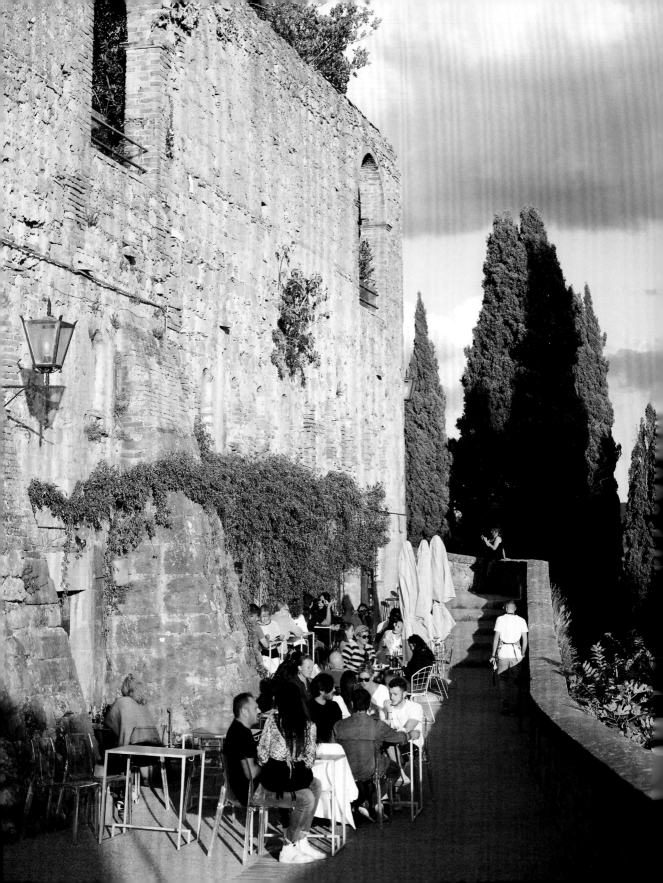

When and Where Italians Eat

I have spent more years than I care to think about grabbing food on the go as I travel for work. The meals available on a television set are rarely well balanced. And when you've been running around all day and then crawl home exhausted in the evening, the temptation to get takeout can be hard to resist. When you are young, you seem to be able to get away with a fast-food existence. Then, one day, you acquire a muffin top over your jeans, dimples in your thighs and the makings of a second chin. Where did these horrors come from? We can run our hearts out at the gym, but unless we adopt a nutritious, balanced diet, those packets of processed food will come back to bite us in that not-so-firm bum.

I've learned so much from the Italians about why they seem trimmer, fitter and healthier. For starters, they simply eat food that is good for them. They consume a diet that is mostly plant-based, rarely eating processed food and limiting meat and fish. There's very little snacking. And it is also *how* they eat: taking the time and effort to cook even if they are alone, and as much as possible making food preparation and mealtime a social occasion amongst friends.

Prima Colazione The First Meal

Breakfast in Italy breaks the mould of what we have been told should be the most important meal of the day. *Prima colazione* is puzzling to many outsiders. Most Italians will enter a bar and order an espresso or a cappuccino, which is basically an espresso with foamed milk. They'll choose a small pastry, stand at the counter and munch it down whilst having a quick chat with those around them, then race off to start their day. No smoothies, bowls of yogurt or high-protein eggy dishes. How on earth do they call this quick, sweet bite a first *meal*? Well, Jacky tells me it is all about balance. The Italians eat little sweet food during the rest of the day, seldom consume desserts except on special occasions and don't go for sugary snacks. Soda is a rare treat.

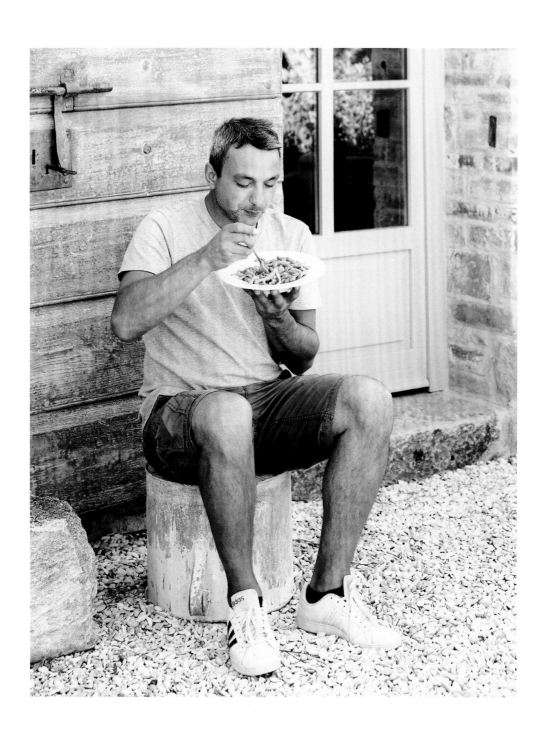

Pranzo The Main Meal of the Day

After their light but high-carb breakfast, Italians dive into *pranzo*, a nutritious lunch being their most important meal of the day. They flock to restaurants or go home to Mamma for a homemade lunch consisting of several courses, followed by a nap. The ritual is a romantic one, to be sure, and perhaps not as common as in the past, now that parts of Italy have become as hectic as the rest of the world. But even those who don't have time for a sit-down meal and instead just grab a slice of pizza wouldn't think of eating it at their desk.

In rural Tuscany, however, the full two- to three-hour lunch remains the status quo.

Aperitivo An Hour that Excites the Appetite

When I first arrived in Italy, I found it challenging to keep up with all the foodie delights and still avoid becoming a ball of lard. I was forever at events, parties or restaurants where it was normal to stuff yourself with every enticing mouthful. Or so it seemed at first. Observing more closely, it was clear that the elegant Italian women made their choices carefully from an array of vegetable side dishes rather than the whole hog—or at least the whole prosciutto. Aha!

Then came my lesson in the *aperitivo*. The character of these pre-dinner drinks and nibbles varies from region to region, but one of the intentions is to stimulate the taste buds for dinner. It's kind of like a cocktail hour, but is so much more than discounted drinks and bowls of peanuts. It is a time to unwind and people-watch while sipping a Campari and soda or a thirst-quenching beer and nibbling on the dozens of different bite-sized samples bars pride themselves on serving free. (Yes, it's fine to eat as much as you want, as long as you buy a drink, which I can always manage.) The large bars in hotels and fashionable areas of a city offer a banquet of small bites of bread with a variety of toppings, bowls of olives, stuffed anchovies, slices of salami made with fennel seeds, chunks of pecorino cheese, deep-fried cauliflower florets, fresh artichokes and sun-dried tomatoes, plus any particular regional specialities. The local village bars are a little more modest with their offering of nibbles, but there is always something delicious.

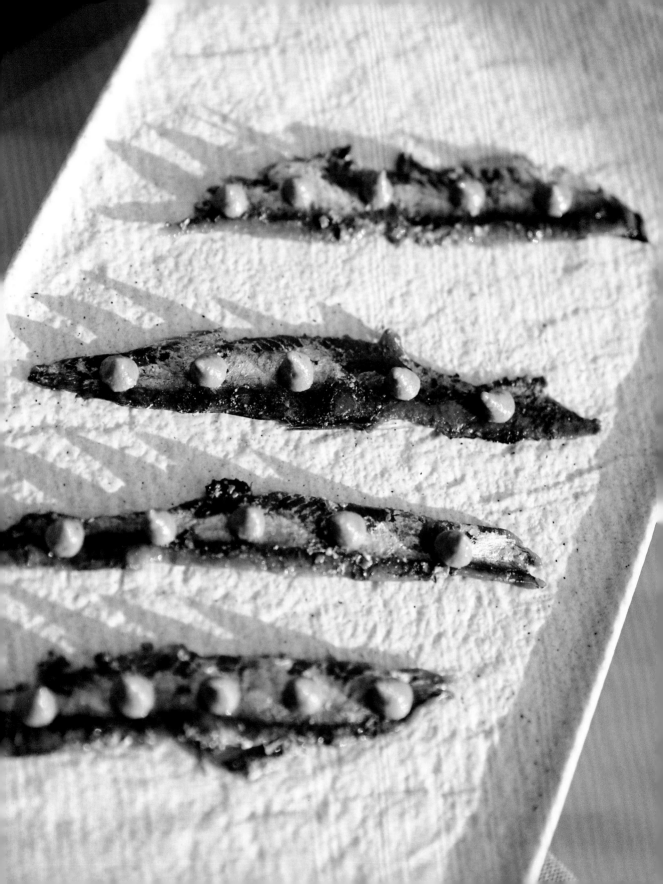

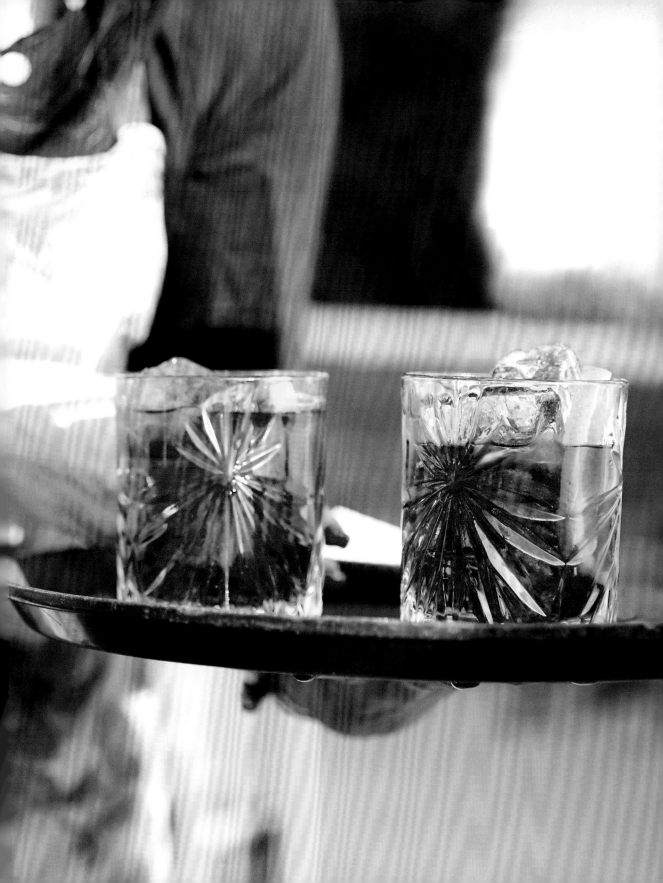

JACKY SAYS

There's a rhyme and reason to the traditional Italian way of eating. Instead of a plate of a starchy food alongside meat and vegetables, try a small amount of pasta or rice first, which will begin to fill you up. Eating slowly allows the brain to catch up with the stomach. Chewing food well is important because digestion begins in the mouth, especially for carbohydrates.

There is nothing wrong with having the occasional smoothie as a replacement meal, but if you make it a habit, your digestive system may become confused and stop producing enough enzymes to break down food. This, in turn, can lead to bloating, heartburn and acid reflux. When we chew, we break food down mechanically, helping the stomach process everything before the food moves into the small intestine, whose job it is to absorb most of the nutrients. If you miss out on the chewing stage by consuming too many liquid meals, that's when problems may arise.

One day, a beautiful local winemaker told me that she rarely eats dinner—she just nibbles her way through the free *aperitivo* in her local bar. Talk about light bulbs going off! Now, unless we are entertaining, this will often be our evening meal. For the price of a drink, you can eat like a king.

Bringing the *aperitivo* tradition home is also delightful. Invite friends around to your place for a drink. Serve good-quality bread with a variety of toppings and a bowl of olives. Pile chopped tomatoes onto toast, add a little olive oil, coarse salt and a few leaves of basil and, wow, you have bruschetta. You can have fun with friends—lots of them—at a much more reasonable cost than providing a full dinner. If conversation lags, then the *aperitivo* comes to an end as planned at seven or eight, but if a good time is being had by all, just keep adding to the spread of tasty treats and the evening can progress without you having to hunker down in the kitchen.

Cena Time for Dinner

The evening meal, *cena*, is generally light. But sometimes, the *aperitivo* is just a warm-up for a full-on feast. When you first get the chance to join the festivities of an Italian communal dinner, you will understand the meaning of being in heaven. You gawk, you inhale, you taste—and you never want to leave the table. The dinner is a marathon of courses, beginning with an *antipasto*, or appetizer. Once your appetite is whetted, the first course, *il primo*—a pasta or rice dish—is served. Then *il secondo* is proudly paraded down the table, the second course of succulent meat or fish or both. There will be numerous side dishes of vegetables (*il contorno*) and roasted, boiled or fried potatoes. If you are not bursting at the seams after all that, dig in to *la dolce*, piles of fresh fruit, cakes, pastries, puddings and pies. And the finale? The pouring of a *digestivo*, a sweet alcoholic drink partnered with homemade biscotti.

It's All in the Portions

I have dieted on and off since I first went in front of a camera. I'd have run a mile if the Italian way of eating had ever been suggested to me during my modelling days. Pizza, pasta and olive oil? Oh, the horrors. Yet the more time I spend in this country, the healthier I feel. Obesity is uncommon around our villages, and as I learned to emulate the lifestyle, my fear of delicious food evaporated.

So what's the secret? It's not only a balanced diet, including good-quality, locally grown, organic ingredients, but also, crucially, portion size. When I mentioned the sweet pastry that Italians typically eat for breakfast, I should have pointed out that it is tiny, at most half the size of a North American croissant, and made with less sugar. Pasta is enjoyed daily by just about everyone in Italy, but the portions are small. The meals at the villa are four courses, but the size of the servings is a fraction of what guests from North America are used to. The cooked portions of pasta or rice are the size of a small fist. A portion of meat or fish is the size of half a hand. Eating this way allows us to revel in a long meal in good company, and we get to taste everything but not overdo it.

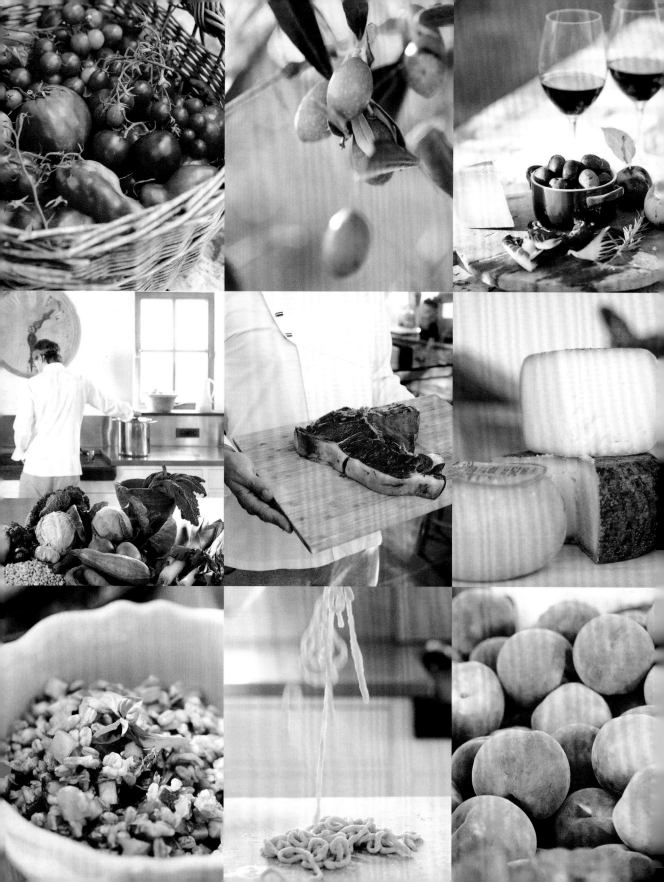

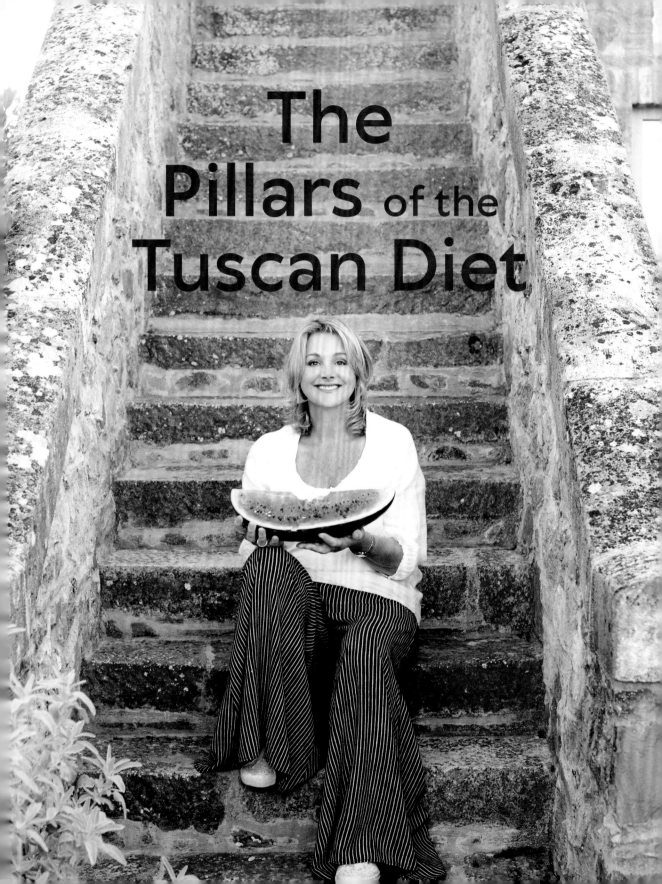

The Pillars of the Tuscan Diet

MANY YEARS HAVE GONE BY SINCE I HAD MY FIRST TRUE Tuscan meal. Hans and I were tourists and had wandered through the massive gates of the fortress town of Montalcino to find a spot of lunch after realizing we were too early to check into our bed and breakfast. The place was deserted—not a soul in sight except for one bent old lady moving slowly in front of us. I think she may have been the smallest adult I have ever seen. We caught up to her easily and asked if there was a restaurant nearby. She placed her warm, wrinkled hand in mine and, like an eager child, pulled us around a corner. We walked through what seemed like the side of someone's home into a covered garden bursting with gnarled wisteria vines. Under the ceiling of purple blossoms were tables crammed with lunchtime revellers. Our new friend pushed us onto a bench at the end of a long table already full of people devouring their meal. The server offered no menu, instead delivering two glass tumblers of red wine and two bowls of steaming traditional pici pasta with a tomato sauce that rendered us speechless. We had stumbled upon heaven.

Tuscan food elicits as much adoration as its artistic heritage. With its origins in the diet of rural peasants, it is a cuisine evolved from necessary resourcefulness. Today, while the locally grown produce features more abundance in choice, farming and cooking methods remain faithful to their roots. The food of the nobility came from the rich cities, but it is the farm table, oblivious to modern trends, that has proved to be the key to longevity, proving the wisdom in the adage "Eat like a peasant, not a rich man."

The essential concepts of Tuscan cuisine are similar to the way our grandparents once cooked. Nothing goes to waste, poor cuts of meat are cooked extensively to extract the nutrients, and the summer harvest is bottled, jarred, dried or pickled for the colder months ahead. Food is not "mucked about with," as my own granny would say, and there are few long and complicated cooking instructions. There is so much to be learned from Tuscan food traditions that counteracts the "noise" of today's diets with time-tested wisdom.

The pillars of the Tuscan diet are plenty of fresh vegetables, a little fruit, beans and grains, complemented by a small amount of dairy, meat and fish and the queen herself, olive oil.

Eat Your Veggies

Any way you slice it, Italians are passionate about vegetables. The long growing season in Tuscany nourishes its people throughout the year. In winter, cavolo nero, an Italian kale variety with long, undulating black leaves, is a staple packed with vitamins and many minerals. Violet-hued artichokes are abundant and are used in all kinds of sauces. Beets, earthy and sweet, are a favourite, and Tuscans use the whole plant, sautéing the stems and leaves with olive oil and garlic. The versatile leek and the weird, knobbly root celeriac are common inclusions in winter soups, and even certain varieties of lettuce grow throughout the cold months.

The arrival of the beloved spring bounty announces the end of the long, dark days of winter. Everyone celebrates, restaurant doors are flung open and the markets explode in a rainbow of goodies. First, peas bounce in with their edible young shoots, then quickly on their heels come fat, broad fava beans, so sweet they are often eaten raw during an *aperitivo*. Asparagus season leads us into summer, which gifts us with the versatile zucchini, countless types of tomatoes, and eggplant (*melanzano*) in shades ranging from black to baby blue, white and even striped. Mushrooms show up as fall muscles in and are paraded around the market stalls like a miracle—we have waited so long! While less tasty cultivated varieties are available in the supermarkets year-round, foraged porcini, with their meaty flavour and texture take centre stage in kitchens up and down the country from October to December.

All of these foods are seasonal and local. Too much of the same thing can sometimes drive one batty, but just as you think you cannot swallow another green bean, the next choice of vegetable pokes its head into the kitchen. There is no better example of the challenges of plenitude than zucchini. It grows with a fervour from July to well into September, and like a cuckoo squatting in another bird's nest, it will invade the garden if not controlled with a firm hand. It's hardly the most exciting of foods, but this is where the genius of the Italian cook is on full display. First, the young zucchini flowers are poached, stuffed, fried, grilled or scattered with artistic flare on pizzas. Then the rather tasteless vegetable is cut into chunks,

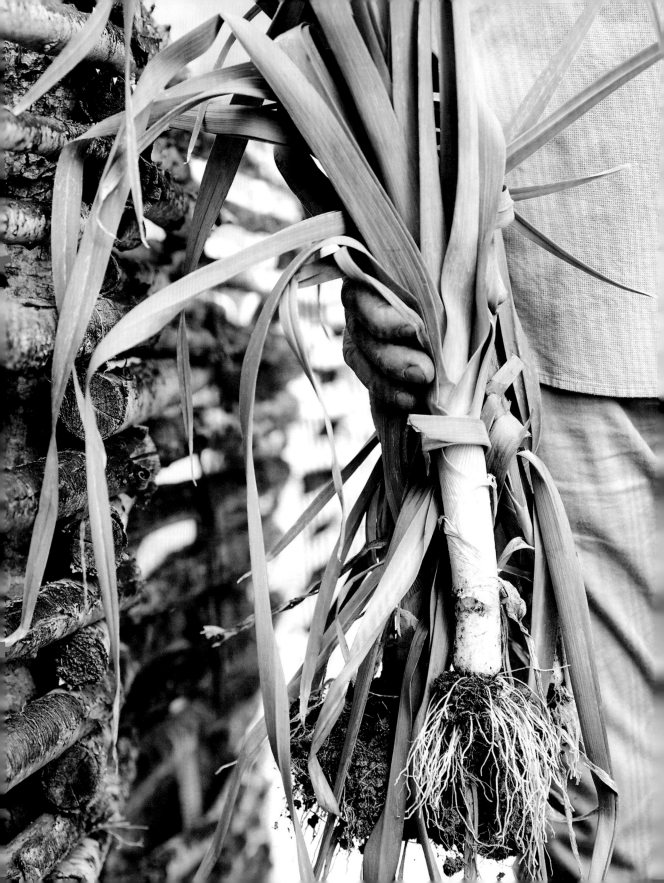

JACKY SAYS

Try to buy organic vegetables wherever possible. Even though all the pesticides in modern-day farming are said to be safe for human consumption, I prefer organic because the chemical companies often test pesticides individually but not in conjunction with the other pesticides, food additives and medications that individuals may be ingesting. You want to avoid a possible buildup of foreign chemicals and toxins in your body. Plus, organic veggies just taste better.

As for vegetable cooking methods, steaming is the way to go, as it does the least damage to the nutrients. When you boil your vegetables, the nutrients leach out into the water. While grilling is popular in the summer, you need to be cautious about crisping and burning. Research has shown that when starch-dense foods and meats are cooked at very high temperatures, or are burnt, the resulting char is linked to known carcinogens. Italians tend not to deep-fry but instead sauté over low heat with good olive oil, stock and seasonings. That makes sense, because it is high heat that destroys the goodness in our food.

rounds or strips and is boiled, puréed, marinated, stuffed, sautéed, steamed, fried, baked or thrown on the grill.

The Tuscans waste little, especially from the garden. At the villa we go through mounds of vegetables daily. We eat up most of the plant, and what leaves and peelings are left, we throw into a pot and simmer with a little salt, so we always have vegetable stock on hand. It takes no time and costs absolutely nothing. What we don't use right away, we freeze.

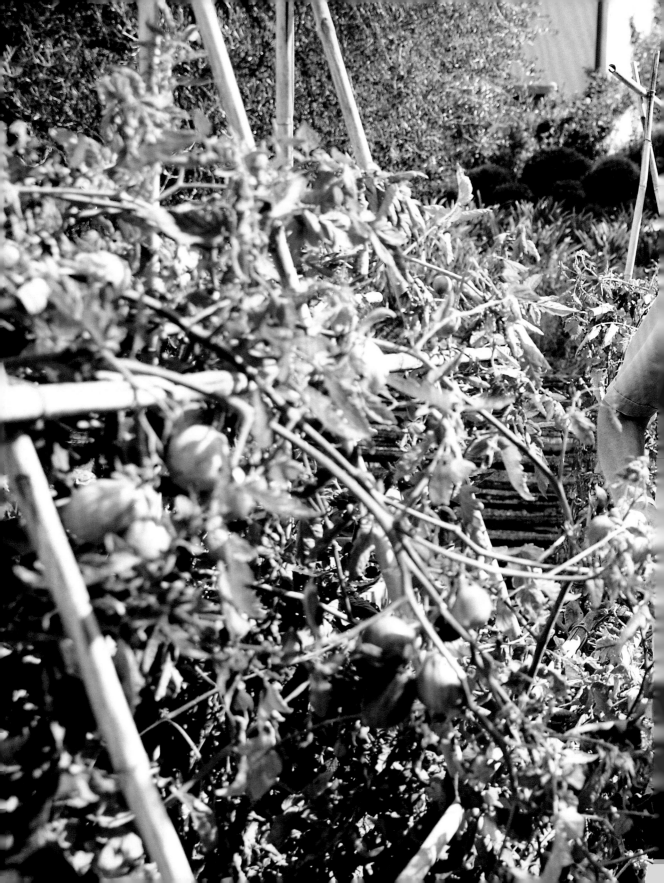

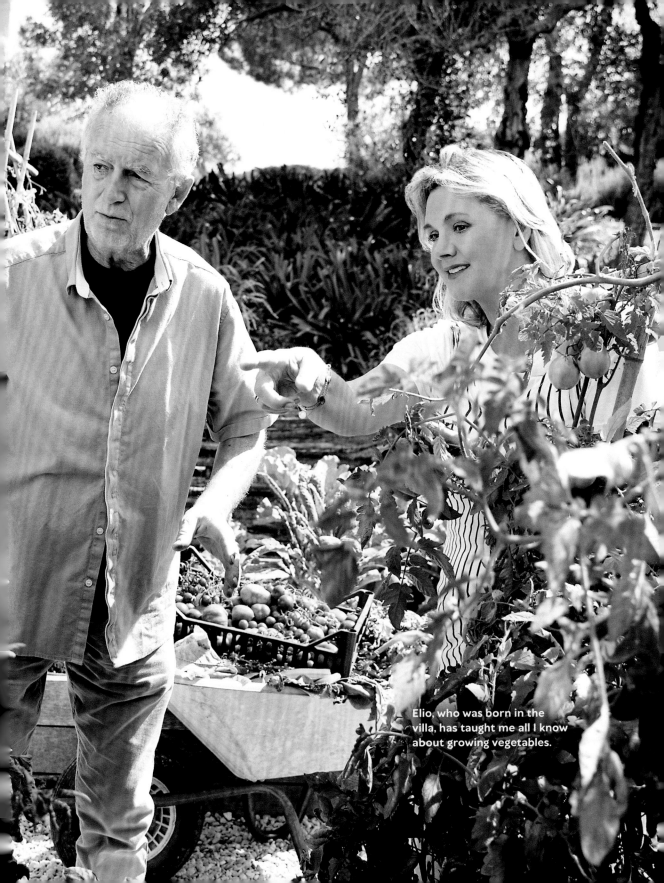

Elio, who was born in the villa, has taught me all I know about growing vegetables.

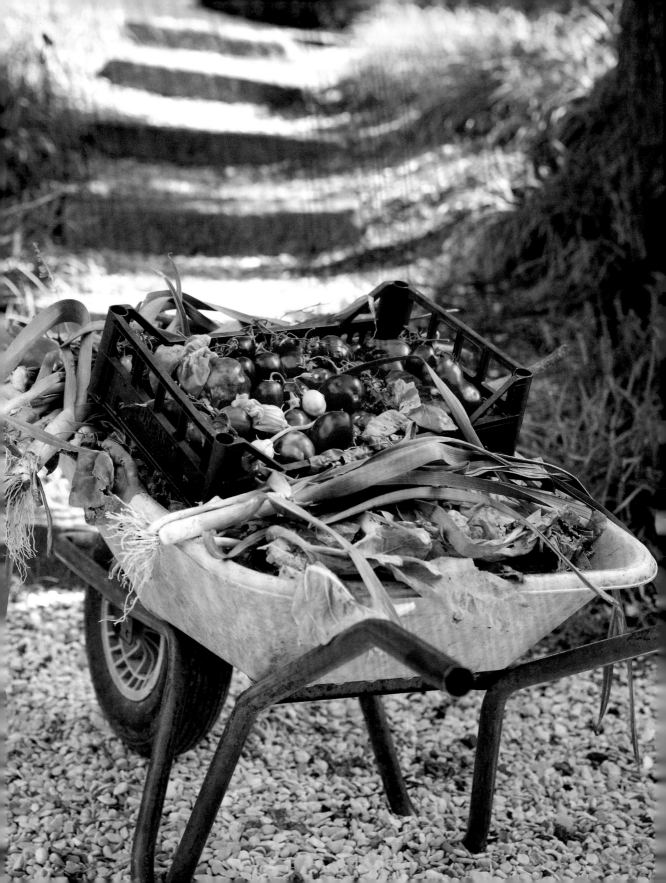

The Kitchen Garden

The vegetable garden, *l'orto*, is indispensable to the way of life here. If people own some land, they will create a kitchen garden; if not, many will have a small plot somewhere nearby in the community. Above our property is a half acre owned by Franco and Renata, an elderly couple who live in the village. For fifty years Franco has grown enough vegetables and fruit to feed his large family, and the chickens and rabbits he raises supply their protein.

But for anyone who tends a garden, it is more than just the produce that matters—it is being in touch with the land, the sensation of seeing your own labour flourish, an escape from the stress of everyday life and an opportunity to bond with like-minded others over the state of the weather and the size of your zucchini. Our own kitchen garden is a feast for the eyes all year long, and its bounty feeds everyone at the villa.

I always loved to get dirty as a child. In my garden I am in my happy place, digging and planting and being part of the dance of nature. I'm often joined by dear Elio, who has taught me when to plant and prune. He is the one in charge, and he nurtures the garden daily. For me, the sheer joy of seeing family, and even guests, harvesting for the next meal, completely content in the moment, is paradise.

In England we have allotments, slices of carefully tended land for non-commercial use, and I remember, as a girl, watching men pottering away while chatting alongside other gardeners. Today, all over the world, the community garden is having a remarkable resurgence. Flat rooftops and unused pieces of land are being repurposed as shared urban vegetable gardens. Growing our own organic produce is such a marvellous way for our children to learn about where their food comes from, and is a valuable way to bring families and communities together. It's an inspiring trend that deserves to keep on thriving.

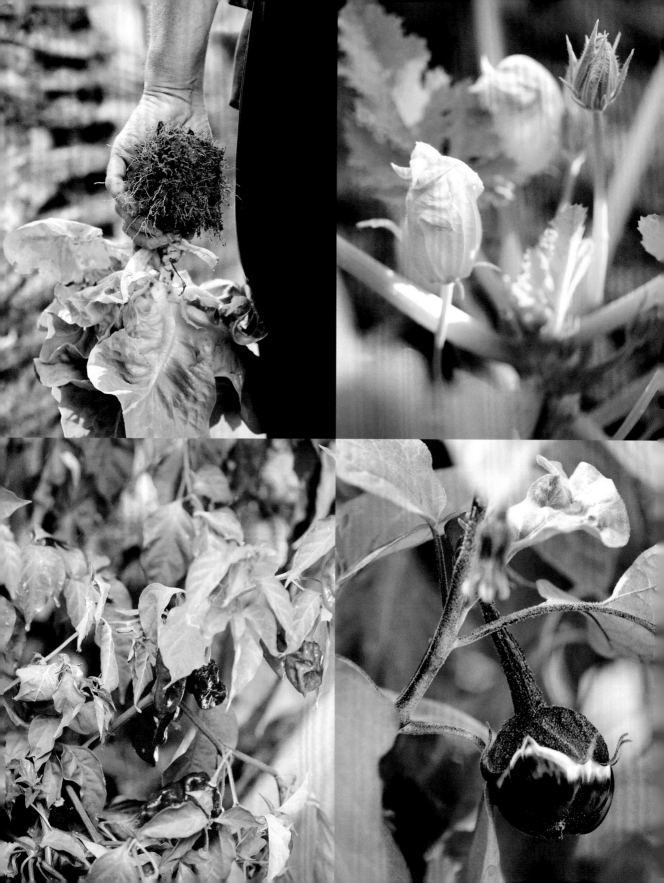

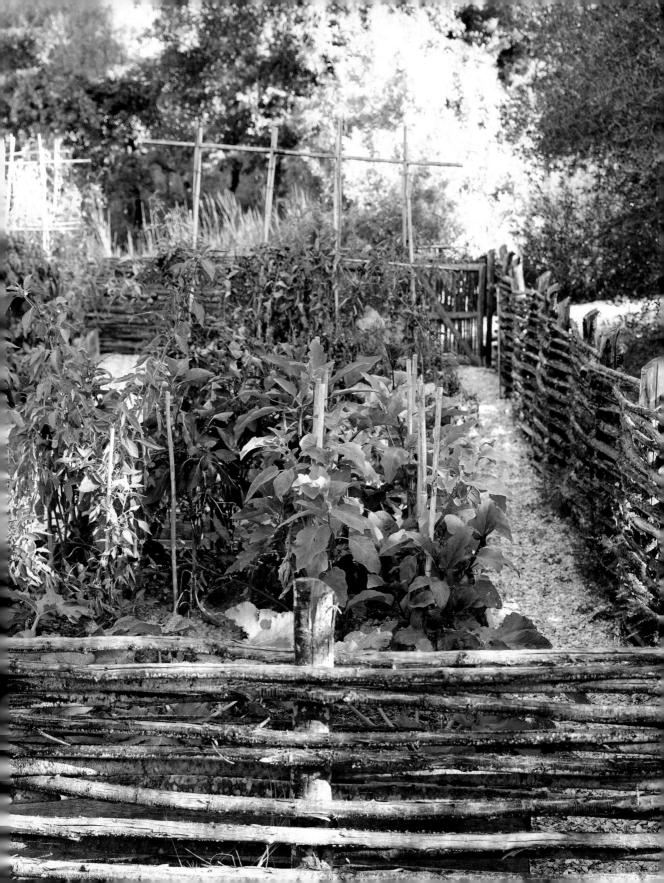

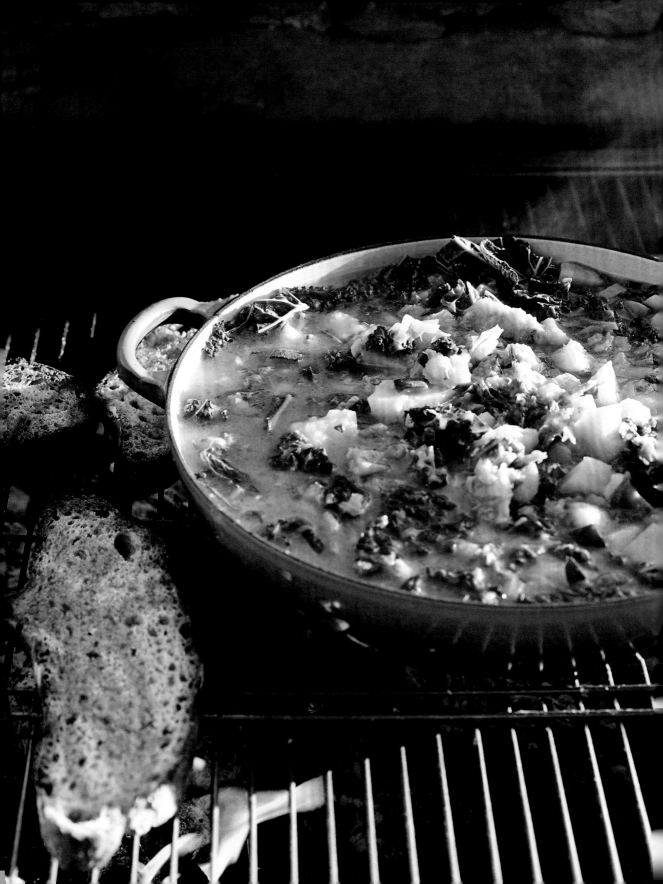

RIBOLLITA

Ribollita, which means "reboiled," is a humble, frugal and tasty meal-in-a-bowl made with leftover vegetables from last night's dinner or whatever scraps you have in your fridge. White cannellini beans are added to the vegetables, along with stock and tomatoes. The Tuscan tradition is to add stale bread at the end of cooking, but we prefer to pile the thick soup onto coarse whole wheat toast and top with a drizzle of olive oil.

¼ cup extra virgin olive oil

1 large carrot, peeled and diced

1 large onion, diced

1 stalk celery, diced

2 zucchini, diced

1 potato, peeled and diced

4 cups vegetable stock
(see recipe, page 209)

3 large pinches of salt

1½ cups julienned black kale, savoy cabbage, chard or combination of all three (any kale and cabbage in season will do!)

2 cups rinsed drained canned cannellini (white kidney) beans or 1½ cups dried beans, soaked overnight and then cooked (see note)

1 teaspoon freshly ground pepper

TO SERVE:

¼ cup chopped fresh parsley

¼ cup chopped fresh basil

Extra virgin olive oil, for drizzling

Freshly grated Parmesan cheese (optional)

8 slices Tuscan bread
(or other crusty bread)

In a large pot, over medium heat, warm the olive oil. Add the carrot, onion and celery. Cook, stirring occasionally, for a few minutes, until softened, then add the zucchini and potato. Add the stock, then the salt, stirring to combine. Increase the heat and bring to a boil, then lower the heat and simmer, partially covered, for about 40 minutes, until the vegetables are cooked. Add the kale, beans and ground pepper, and continue to simmer, uncovered, for 20 to 30 minutes, until the kale is al dente.

To serve: Ladle the soup into bowls and sprinkle with parsley and basil, drizzle with olive oil and, if desired, add a sprinkle of grated Parmesan. Add the bread to the soup. (Or serve the bread up as toast and add a dollop of the thick soup to each bite.)

NOTE: To cook dried cannellini beans, place them in a large bowl and add 4½ cups of cold water (for the amount of beans in this recipe, or use 3 cups of water for every 1 cup of beans). Cover and let soak for about 10 hours or overnight. (For these and any dried beans, it's a good idea to add a tablespoon of apple cider vinegar, which neutralizes the phytates, natural plant enzymes that inhibit the absorption of minerals.) Drain and rinse the beans, then return them to the pot, cover generously with fresh water and bring to a boil. Lower the heat and simmer gently until soft, about 1 hour. Drain and use immediately or let cool before storing.

The Fabulous Radicchio

Pliny the Elder, a commander during the early days of the Roman Empire, was also a naturalist. He wrote about radicchio, praising its many medical properties. Signore Pliny was definitely on to something: radicchio (part of the chicory family) contains good levels of antioxidants and plenty of vitamin K, wonderful for bone strength and healthy blood clotting. High in fibre, it also provides many minerals and some B vitamins, and its natural bitterness is good for our digestion.

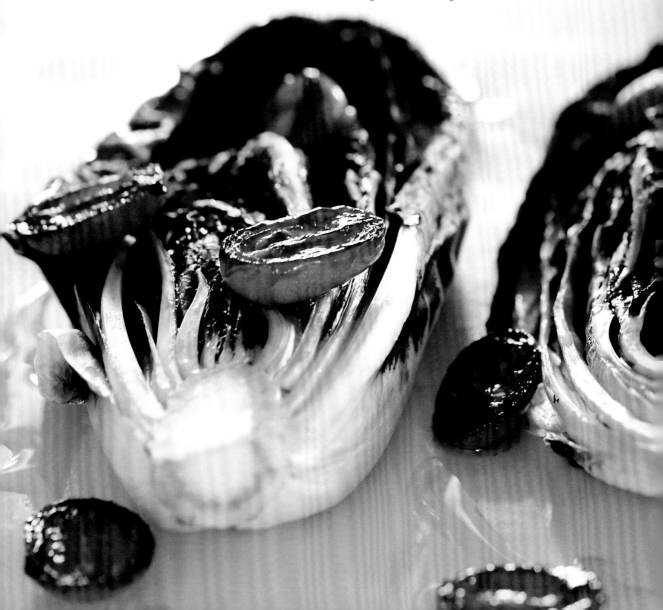

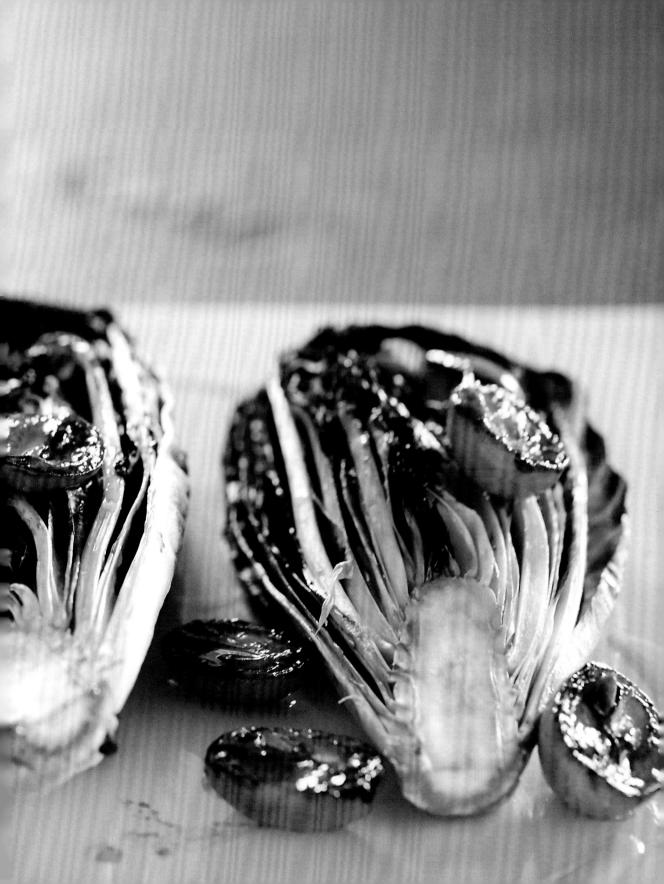

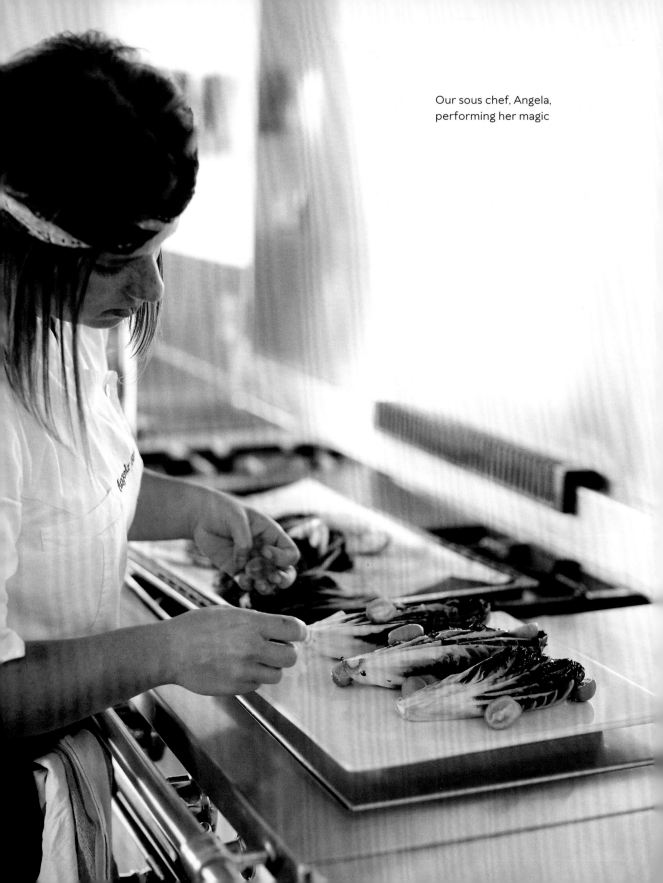

Our sous chef, Angela,
performing her magic

ROASTED RADICCHIO

We eat a great deal of radicchio at the villa—it grows abundantly and quickly in our kitchen garden. It's tasty as an element of a crisp and cool summer salad, but is even more popular as a warm dish. In the late spring, cherries perfectly complement the vegetable's natural bitterness. If cherries aren't in season, Chef Francesco uses sweet little tomatoes and a sprinkling of crumbled feta cheese. Served with some Tuscan bread on the side, it's the perfect lunch.

4 heads of radicchio, external leaves removed

Juice of 1 lemon

¼ cup balsamic vinegar

¼ teaspoon coarse salt

Freshly ground pepper

¼ cup extra virgin olive oil

A couple of handfuls halved yellow and/or red grape tomatoes (or pitted fresh sweet cherries)

½ cup crumbled feta cheese (optional)

Preheat the oven to 350°F (180°C).

If the radicchio heads are round, cut each one in half through the core end, then cut each half into three wedges. If the heads are elongated, slice each in half lengthwise.

For the vinaigrette, in a medium bowl, whisk together the lemon juice, vinegar, salt and pepper. Whisk in the olive oil, little by little, until completely blended.

On a baking sheet lined with parchment paper, spread the tomatoes in a single layer. Place the radicchio on top (as it cooks, the radicchio will absorb some of the sweet juices). Pour the vinaigrette evenly over the radicchio. Roast for 12 minutes, until the radicchio begins to wilt. Flip the tomatoes and radicchio over and roast for another 8 minutes.

Serve family-style on a large serving dish or wooden platter. Sprinkle with feta cheese, if using.

Praise the Tomato, Both the Perfect and the Misshapen

It is no exaggeration to say Italy loves tomatoes. Robust and versatile, they're a go-to throughout the year. Picked from the garden and eaten fresh during the summer, the bountiful crop is frozen, dried or bottled and stored to make sauces and soups in the winter months.

If I ask you to envision a moment in your childhood related to the tomato, you might remember being perched at the kitchen table in front of a warming bowl of Campbell's tomato soup—at least, that was my experience! My mum would garnish ours with soldiers of sliced buttered toast. The combination is the taste of my childhood.

Botanically the tomato is a fruit, but it is prepared and consumed like a vegetable. There is little relationship between the flavour and nutrients of the freshly picked garden varieties and their supermarket cousins, which are bred to a perfectly uniform shape and size, picked immature and unripe, then transported for many miles whilst being sprayed with ethylene gas to transform them from green to dazzling red. Why? Because this artificial standard is what the supermarket owners think customers demand.

Wherever you the live, fresh, robust, locally grown, vine-ripened tomatoes are abundant in markets all summer long. They hang in baskets on patios, grow well in large pots and are abundant in backyards all over the world. This is the time to take a page from the Italians, don an apron, gather some friends, open a bottle of crisp white wine and start prepping tomato sauce for the year ahead. It's a delightful way to spend a Sunday afternoon: chopping and dicing, laughing and gossiping. The tomato plants in our kitchen garden are relentlessly productive, so it's a summer-long activity in Tuscany.

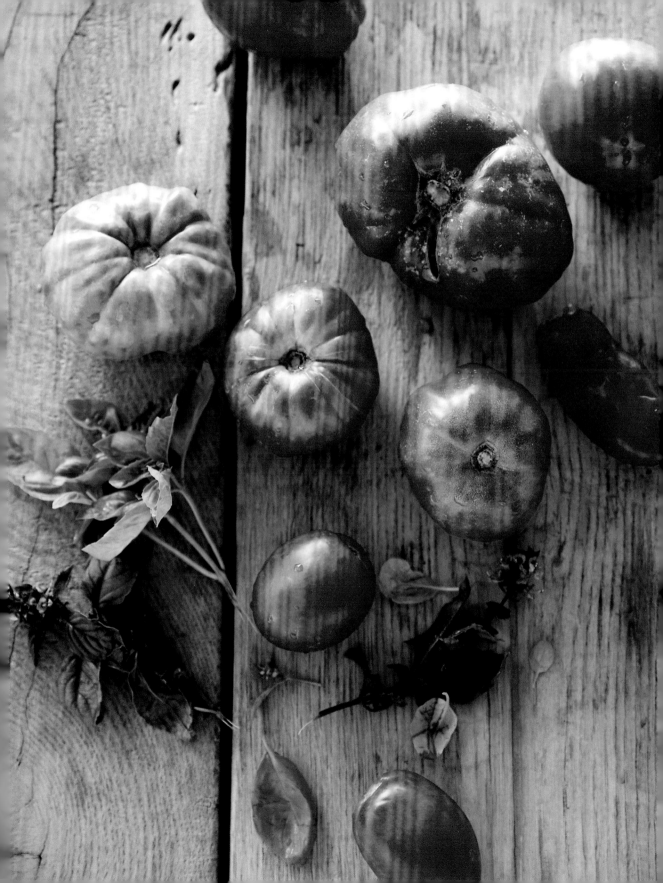

I am a lazy cook. I throw the entire juicy fruit, skins and all, into an enormous pot, then add some chopped onion and celery, rosemary, oregano and garlic and let it bubble away for about an hour. After letting the sauce cool, I ladle portions into zip-lock bags and pop them in the freezer.

The variations are endless. You can whizz the mixture with an immersion blender for a smoother sauce or boil it down further to reduce the liquid for a thicker consistency. Throw in some chili pepper flakes for a spicy version. To intensify the flavour, try oven-roasting the tomatoes instead of boiling them (see page 149). Or make gazpacho instead by whizzing raw tomatoes, garlic, cucumber, bell peppers and onions in a blender.

However I cook my tomatoes, my only challenge is remembering to label the results. I'm always a little bemused when I grab a bag from the freezer—is it a raw tomato purée or a rich cooked sauce?—but being happily stocked up for the winter is the main thing.

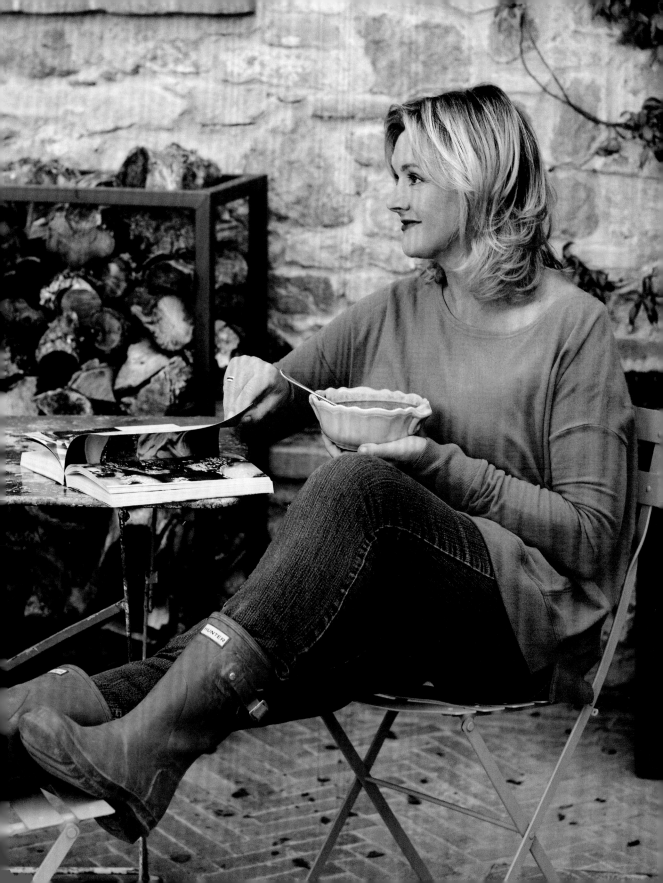

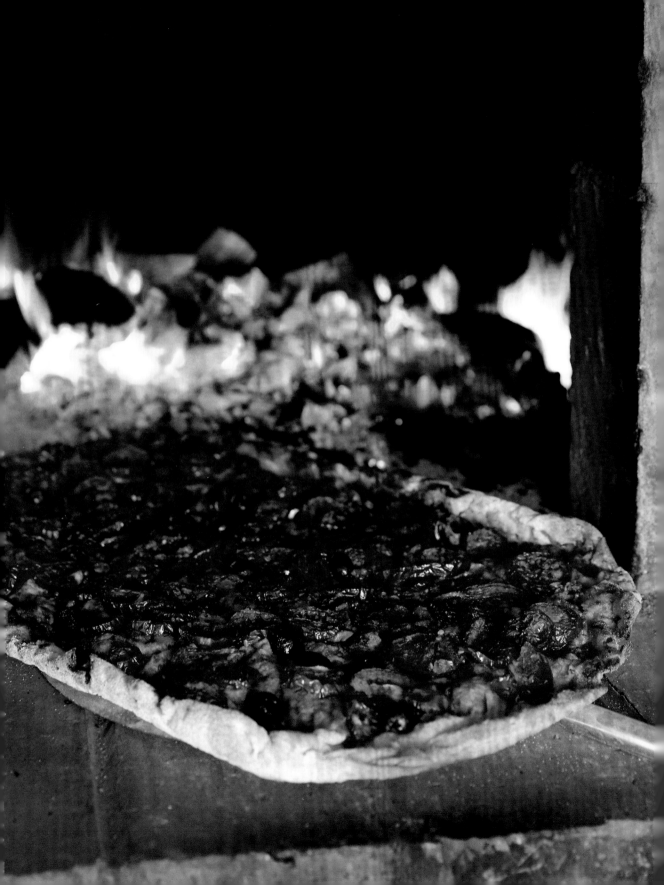

FRESH TOMATO PIZZA

Once street food for the underprivileged citizens of Naples, pizza today needs no introduction, and it's one of our favourites at the villa. We are lucky to still have the original four-hundred-year-old open-air oven on our grounds, where generations have baked bread and pizza. If possible, use local tomatoes, and if there is a vegetarian in the house, replace the anchovies with capers. This recipe uses a tomato-based "paste" with capers for saltiness—it's insane how scrumptious it is—but you can do whatever you like! For example, you could use a pesto-style herb sauce. Get creative!

If you're short on time and don't want to make your own dough, you can buy it ready-made at the supermarket.

ROASTED TOMATOES:

8 Roma (plum) tomatoes, quartered lengthwise

Extra virgin olive oil

Coarse salt

DOUGH:

1 tablespoon salt

1 cup room-temperature water

1½ teaspoons instant yeast or pizza yeast

2⅔ cups all-purpose flour, plus more for sprinkling

Extra virgin olive oil

SAUCE:

¼ cup extra virgin olive oil

¼ cup tomato paste

2 or 3 cloves garlic, crushed

2 tablespoons chopped fresh basil

1 tablespoon chopped fresh oregano

1 teaspoon drained capers

1 teaspoon freshly ground pepper

2 big pinches of salt

TOPPINGS:

¼ large red onion, thinly sliced

Anchovies

Black olives, pitted and halved

A handful of halved cherry tomatoes

Coarse salt

To roast the tomatoes: Preheat the oven to 400°F (200°C) and lightly oil a large baking sheet or roasting pan. Place the tomato quarters, cut side up, in a single layer. Lightly brush each quarter with olive oil and sprinkle with coarse salt. Roast for 20 minutes, until the tomatoes have begun to shrink. Lower the temperature to 225°F (110°C) and roast for 1 hour, checking every so often and giving the tomatoes a stir to make sure nothing is burning and they are roasting evenly. Set the tomatoes aside.

(If making ahead, you can let them cool and then refrigerate them in an airtight container for up to 2 days.)

To make the dough: In a small bowl, dissolve the salt thoroughly in the room-temperature water. Add the yeast and let sit for 5 minutes. Stir with a fork until mixed.

In a large bowl, combine the flour and the yeast mixture, using a pinching motion with your fingers to incorporate the liquid. The mixture will seem a bit dry and shaggy. Turn the fully combined mixture out onto a floured surface and knead for 5 minutes, until smooth.

Lightly oil a large bowl and place the dough in it. Cover with a tea towel and let rise, at room temperature, for 2 hours or until dough has doubled in size.

To make the sauce: Place all of the sauce ingredients in a blender or a food processor fitted with a steel blade. Blend until thoroughly combined. Set aside.

To make the pizza: Preheat the oven to 500°F (260°C). Lightly oil a large baking sheet.

Flour a surface such as a wooden board or a countertop. Turn out the dough onto the floured surface and flatten slightly, then begin to gently stretch it from underneath, using your hands to gradually tease it out. Once the dough is roughly the size of the baking sheet and of even thickness, place it on the oiled pan and stretch to fit.

Pour the sauce over the dough and spread it evenly over the surface. Place the roasted tomatoes on top of the sauce in an even single layer. Scatter the red onion, anchovies, olives and cherry tomatoes on top. Sprinkle with a little coarse salt. Bake for 8 to 12 minutes or until the bottom of the pizza is nicely browned.

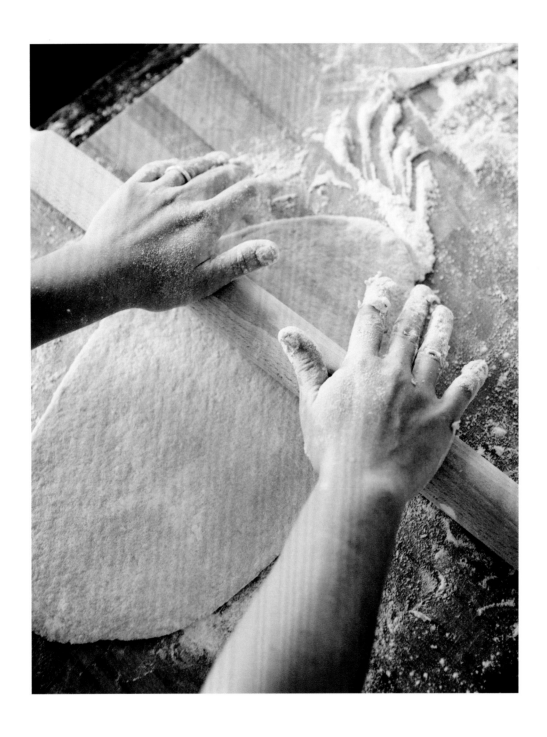

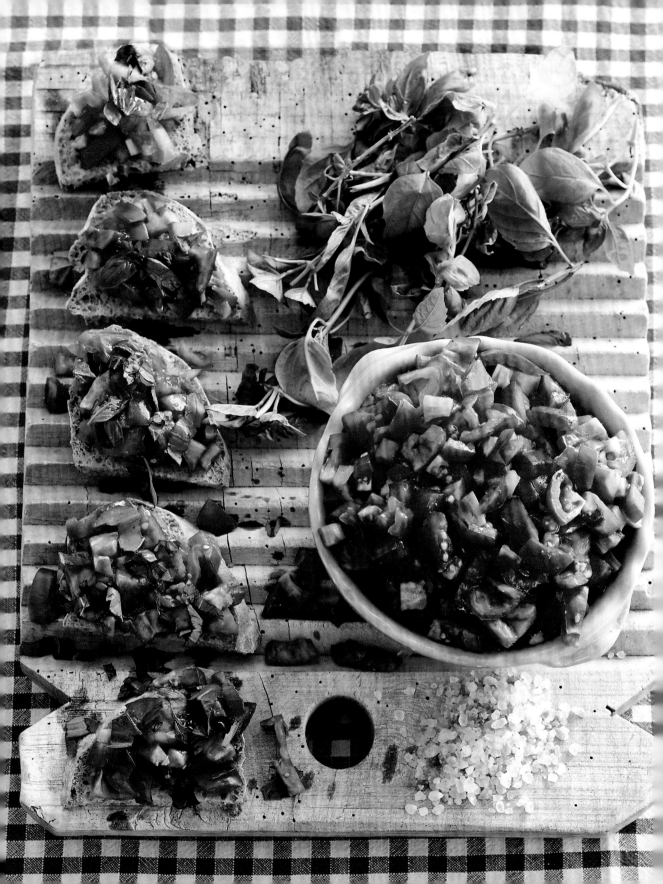

BRUSCHETTA

When the last retreat of the season has come to an end, my hubby and I finally get some alone time—bliss! We are just about "fooded out," and simple is the name of the game. A slice or two of bruschetta for a light supper is divine with a glass of red wine whilst we watch the evening sun slip over the Tuscan hills. You can, of course, get fancy and sprinkle on some roasted pine nuts, crumbled goat cheese or a sliver of prosciutto. Healthy, colourful and delicious, bruschetta is happy food.

6 to 8 slices of your favourite dense, crusty bread (preferably sourdough)
Extra virgin olive oil
2 to 3 cups roughly chopped tomatoes
Handful of fresh basil leaves, shredded
Roasted pine nuts, crumbled goat cheese and/or prosciutto slices (optional)
Coarse salt

Preheat the oven to 425°F (220°C). Place the bread slices on a baking sheet and brush each with olive oil. Bake for 3 minutes. Flip the bread slices over and bake for another 3 minutes, keeping an eye out so they don't burn. Set aside to cool.

Meanwhile, in a large bowl, toss the tomatoes and basil with a good drizzle of olive oil. Once the bread has cooled, generously heap the tomato mixture on top, along with any of the optional toppings. Finally, drizzle with olive oil and sprinkle with coarse salt.

TUSCAN GAZPACHO

Gazpacho originates from Andalusia in southern Spain, but many Mediterranean countries make a version of cold tomato soup. Francesco's recipe is such a hit at the retreats that there is always a crowd around him in the kitchen. The texture of gazpacho varies from thick and chunky to silky smooth, which is how Francesco prepares it. It's elegant and delicate, heavenly on a sizzling summer day. The pickled zucchini garnish gives the soup a tart kick, balancing the sweetness of the tomatoes.

MARINATED ZUCCHINI:

1 tablespoon granulated sugar

1 tablespoon salt

1 cup apple cider vinegar

½ cup extra virgin olive oil

1 large zucchini

GAZPACHO:

1 red bell pepper

1 yellow bell pepper

5 San Marzano or Roma (plum) tomatoes, finely diced

2 cucumbers, peeled, seeded and finely diced

1 large onion, finely diced

1 teaspoon minced garlic

1 teaspoon chili pepper flakes (or 1 small chili pepper, minced)

1 teaspoon freshly ground pepper

Extra virgin olive oil for drizzling

Salt

GARNISH:

Plain yogurt, fresh ricotta cheese or whipping (heavy) cream

Chopped fresh chives

To marinate the zucchini: In a medium bowl, combine the sugar, salt, vinegar and olive oil, whisking for 1 minute. Use a mandoline or vegetable peeler to slice the zucchini lengthwise into very thin ribbons. Place the ribbons in a dish or glass container and pour the marinade over top to cover completely. Cover and refrigerate for 3 to 4 hours.

To make a smooth, velvety gazpacho: Set a small pot of water over high heat and bring to a boil. Add the red and yellow peppers and boil for 4 minutes. Drain and let cool, then remove stems and seeds. In a food processor fitted with a steel blade or a blender, combine the cooled peppers, tomatoes, cucumbers, onion, garlic, chili pepper and pepper. With the machine running, gradually drizzle in olive oil and continue to process until smooth.

Season with salt and pepper to taste. Cover and refrigerate for at least 2 hours, or overnight.

When ready to serve: Ladle the gazpacho into bowls and add a swirl of yogurt and some marinated zucchini to each bowl. Sprinkle with chives.

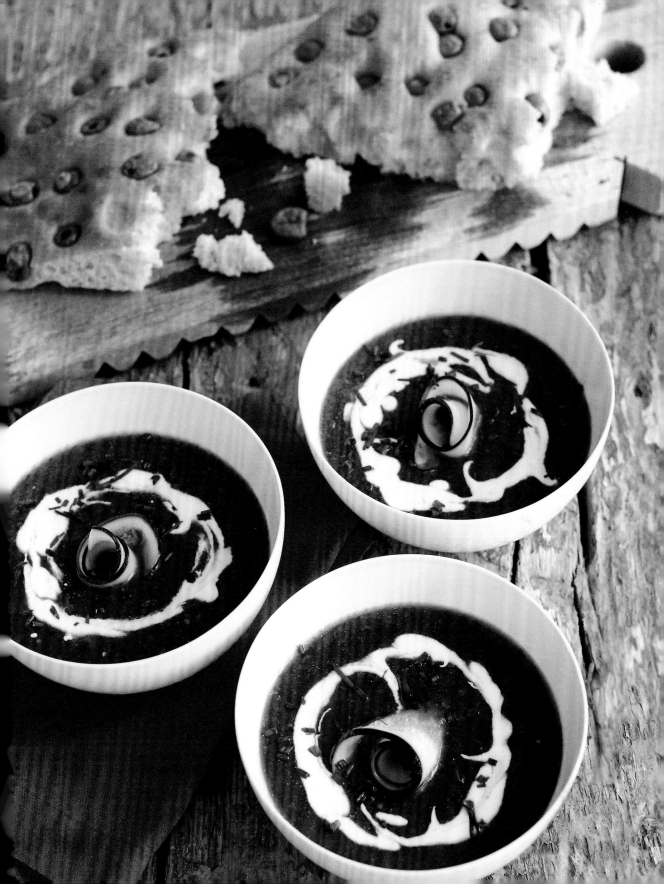

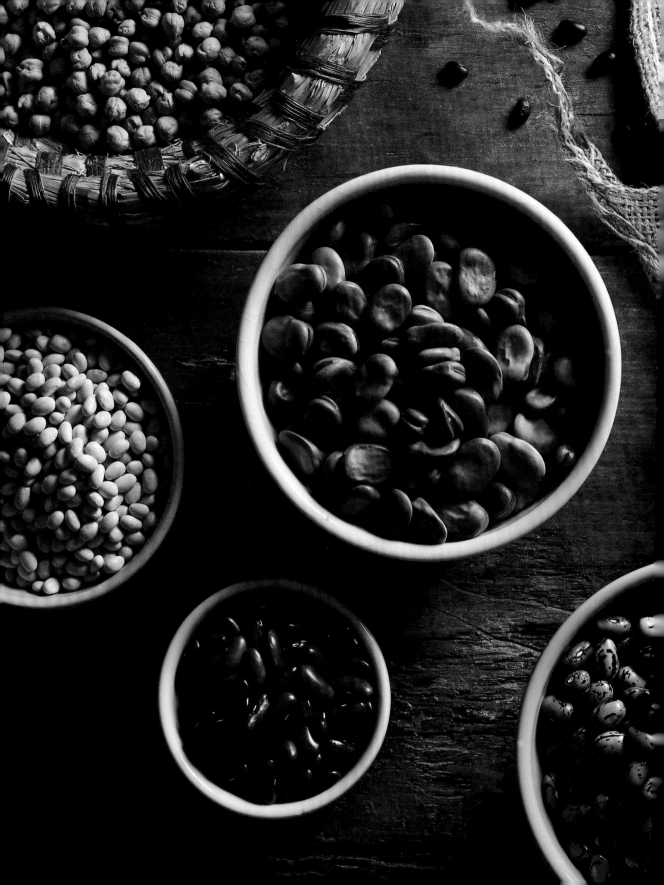

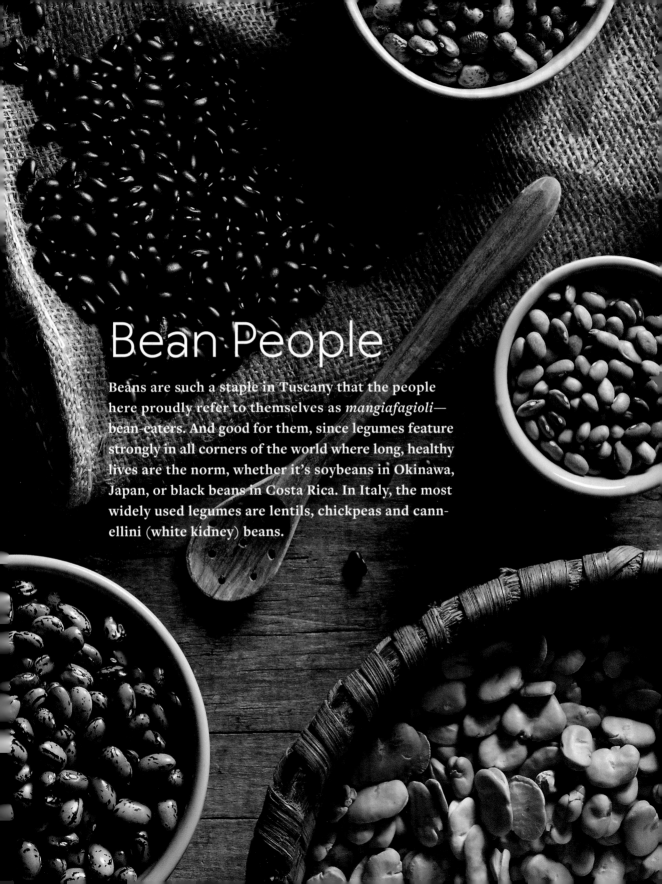

Bean People

Beans are such a staple in Tuscany that the people here proudly refer to themselves as *mangiafagioli*—bean-eaters. And good for them, since legumes feature strongly in all corners of the world where long, healthy lives are the norm, whether it's soybeans in Okinawa, Japan, or black beans in Costa Rica. In Italy, the most widely used legumes are lentils, chickpeas and cannellini (white kidney) beans.

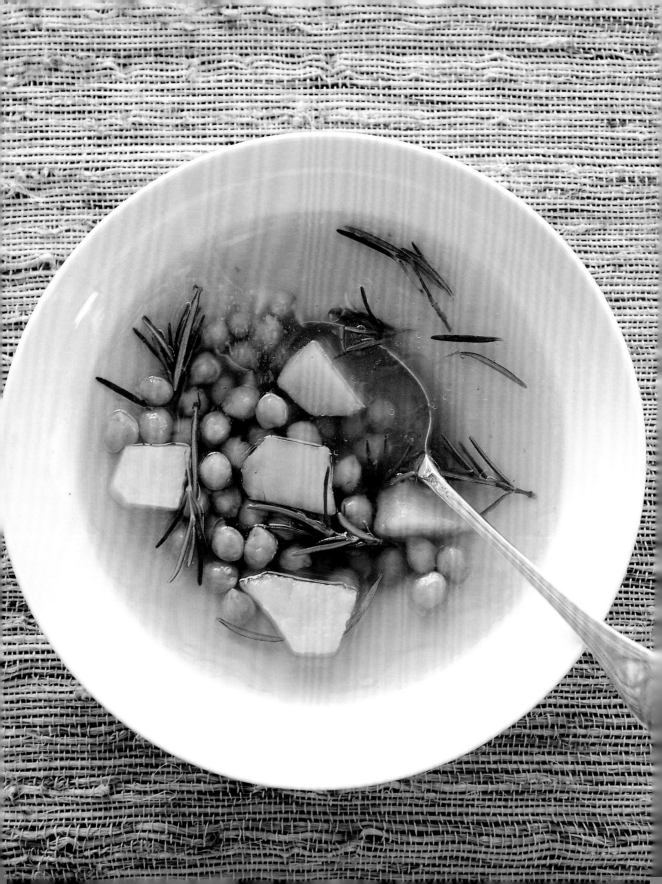

CHICKPEA SOUP

Osteria La Botte Piena is a superb local eatery that serves one of the simplest of dishes: chickpea soup (*zuppa di ceci*). It's such a favourite of mine that I recently followed Elena, the owner, into the kitchen to beg her for the recipe. Here it is: only minutes to make, nutritious and madly cheap.

4 cups vegetable stock (see recipe, page 209) or chicken stock

2 large potatoes (Yukon Gold are ideal, but any will work),
    peeled and cut into 1-inch (2.5 cm) chunks

2 cups cooked chickpeas (or one 540 ml/19 oz can, drained and rinsed)

2 sprigs fresh rosemary, leaves removed from stems

Salt and freshly ground pepper

In a large pot, bring the stock to a boil over high heat. Add the potatoes, lower the heat and simmer for about 20 minutes or until fork-tender.

Set out four soup bowls and evenly distribute the potatoes, chickpeas and rosemary leaves among them. Pour stock into each bowl, dividing evenly, and season to taste with salt and pepper.

> **NOTE:** To cook dried chickpeas, place ⅔ cup chickpeas in a large pot and add 2 cups of cold water (for the amount of cooked beans in this recipe, or use 3 cups of water for every 1 cup of beans). Cover and let soak for about 10 hours or overnight and rinse the chickpeas, then return them to the pot, cover generously with fresh water and bring to a boil. Lower the heat and simmer gently for about 2 hours or until the beans are cooked through but not mushy. Drain and use immediately or let cool before storing.
>
> Beans are about 22 percent protein and 77 percent complex carbohydrate. If you eat a lunch of chickpea soup or bean stew, you won't be longing for a cookie in the middle of the afternoon.

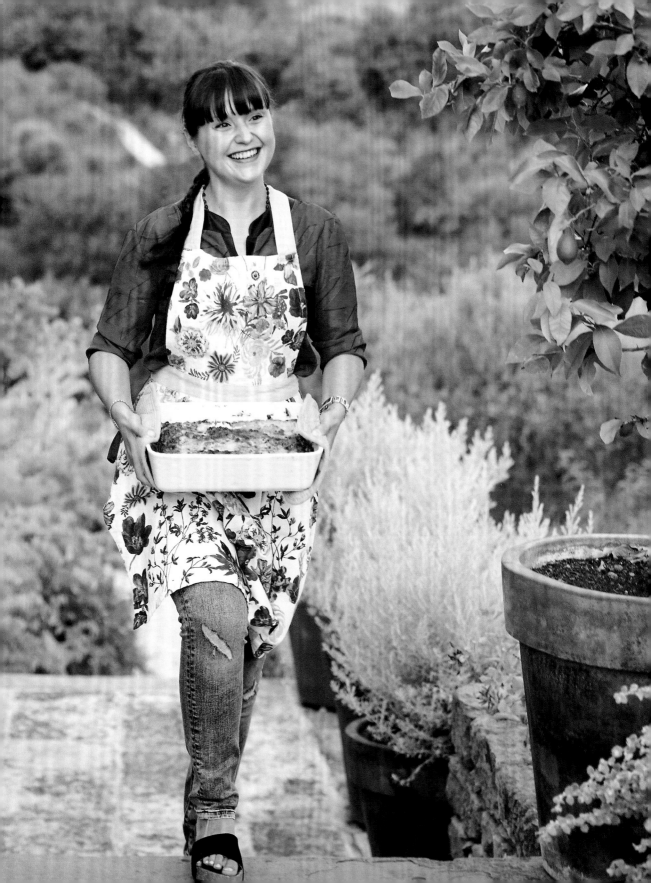

Who's Afraid of the Big Bad Carbs?

Bread, pasta, pizza and pastries in all their mind-boggling varieties are the lifeblood of Italy's population, yet it is rare to see obesity here, so my neighbours must be doing something right.

One of the challenges of spending time in Tuscany has been getting past everything I had previously learned about carbs. *Stay away from bread! Take a pass on pasta!* Starchy carbs have been blamed for many diseases and for our current obesity epidemic, but not all carbs are created equal. Fibre-rich grains are important for good digestion and a healthy gut. It's processed foods, high in refined grains and sugar, that can pile on the pounds and have adverse health effects.

Our guests at Villa Reniella come with countless dietary variables, so Jacky asks them to tell us in advance of any food dislikes and allergies. Each year the list grows longer, especially with those who are gluten-intolerant. The news can bring Chef to his knees—it is not easy to cook for a lactose-free, no-gluten vegan with a nut allergy who loathes vegetables! I am kidding, but believe me we have come close.

I was brought up on sandwiches made with sliced white bread, chips (french fries) and a dollop of ketchup, and I lived to tell the tale. Thankfully, my diet has improved immeasurably, but I do feel we have all gone a bit loopy and bought into the hype of commercial food giants pushing the latest fads in order to sell new products.

For people who truly must avoid gluten, such as those with celiac disease, it is a difficult ongoing battle. Thankfully, researchers continue to dig into the causes of celiac disease and how to treat it. But when our guests tell us they suffer only mild symptoms after consuming gluten, we ask them to give the local pasta and bread a try. They seem to digest it with no issue—and much satisfaction.

Pasta and Bread

The shelves in North American supermarkets are lined with packets of Italian pasta in all shapes and sizes. But look closely: many of the famous Italian brands are actually manufactured in North America and might use a different type of wheat than the same brand in Italy.

Italians have strict laws protecting the production of pasta, including one to maintain nutrient values by using a hard grain—usually semolina produced from durum wheat. This grain contains higher levels of protein than soft grains, making the pasta easier to digest. In addition, the hard grain has a lower glycemic index (GI), meaning it takes longer for the body to convert the carbs into glucose, which in turn allows blood sugar levels to remain stable.

In addition, Italians always cook their pasta al dente, which means "firm to the tooth," or not cooked all the way through. The taste and texture are far better than those of overcooked pasta, and the slight roughness holds the sauce better, but there are nutritional benefits, too: al dente pasta actually has a lower glycemic index.

So if pasta does not usually agree with you, you might be able to chalk it up to the type of wheat or the cooking method. Look for pastas made from durum wheat, keep portions to 1 cup of cooked pasta and cook it al dente. An entire nation cannot be wrong!

When it comes to fresh pasta (*pasta fresca*) or dried pasta (*pasta secca*), neither is considered superior—it is more about the texture and how it holds the sauce. Every Italian will discuss this endlessly. Dried pasta is firmer, so it's perfect for meaty sauces or ragù, while fresh pasta is better for tossing with lighter sauces based on tomatoes or cream. *Pasta fresca* usually contains eggs, but even this can depend on the region of Italy. When Chef Francesco leads the cooking class for our guests, he recounts that during and after the Second World War, when food was scarce, women put aside the precious eggs designated for their pasta-making, saving them for the little ones, who needed the protein. "The future is our children," Chef emotionally proclaims to the class. A tear is always shed.

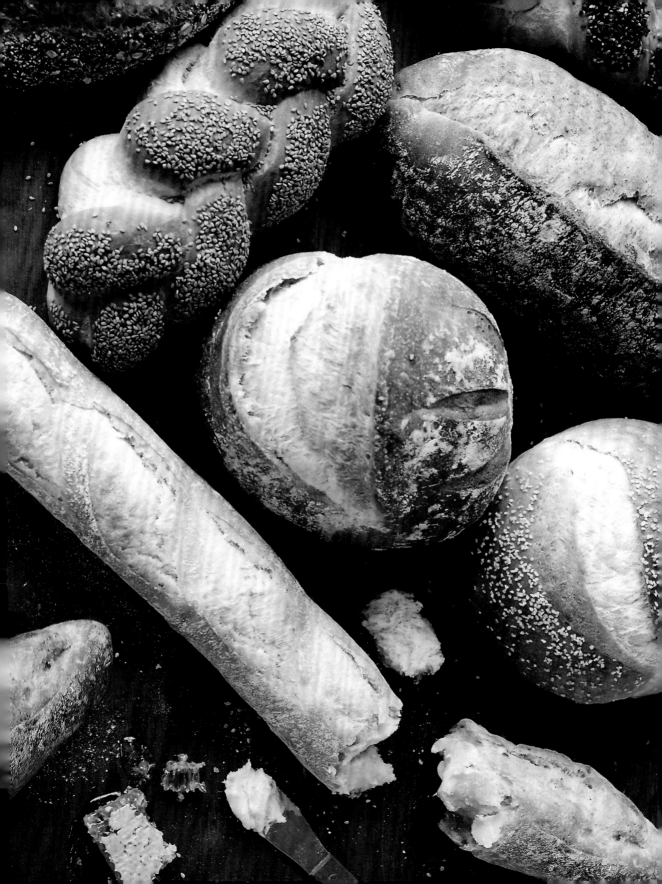

JACKY SAYS

A food's score on the glycemic index tells you how quickly it is converted into sugar once consumed. Every time you eat a food that contains carbohydrate, you experience a change in your blood glucose (sugar) levels. The body's response to carbohydrates can be very different depending on how much sugar the food contains, how processed it is, its fibre content and what other types of food you pair it with. For example, eating protein along with carbs can slow down the body's absorption of sugars.

The nutritional content of bread depends on the type: white, rye, sourdough, whole wheat and all the other varieties under the sun. Essentially, all breads are a source of fibre, starch (carbohydrate) and some protein. Whole wheat varieties contain B vitamins (found in the husk of the grain) and a smidgen of iron. White bread, on the other hand, has had all its goodness stripped out with the removal of the bran, husk and germ (the nutritious centre of the wheat). Mass-manufactured white sandwich breads are fortified with B vitamins, calcium and iron to give them more nutritive value.

A little more on fibre. As a prebiotic, fibre feeds the good bacteria in the large intestine. Eating a balanced diet with plenty of roughage is associated with a lower risk of colon cancer because fibre helps move waste through the digestive system, promoting a regular bowel movement.

Whole grains contain phytochemicals that act as antioxidants, offering a protective role against illnesses including cancer, heart disease and type 2 diabetes. Whole grains also provide vitamins B and E, zinc, potassium and magnesium, as well as a little protein.

Then the pasta-making fun begins. The traditional homemade fresh pasta of our region is pici (see recipe, page 274), a thick, wormlike spaghetti that's ideal for holding a sauce. There are constant laughs around my kitchen island as twenty guests roll and twist their dough into as many shapes as there are personalities.

Like pasta, bread is a foundation food in Italy. Unlike its French cousin, the fluffy, mouth-watering, charming baguette, a Tuscan loaf is not intended to be eaten unadorned. Crostini are made from small round loaves called stinco (a name that has my grown sons giggling each time they order it), cut into slices and piled with toppings: chicken liver spread, bean purée, grilled mushrooms, artichokes or just a drizzle of olive oil and a pinch of coarse salt. Larger pieces of bread are topped with chopped tomatoes (bruschetta) or used as an edible plate when eating ribollita.

Typical Tuscan bread is tasteless, and for a fascinating reason. In Roman times, soldiers were partially paid in salt, then a precious commodity. Their wage, therefore, was called their *sale* (pronounced "sal-ai"), which is the origin of the word *salary*. Salt was also so heavily taxed that people stopped putting it in their bread. And so it remains today—this is a place of traditional grudges. The bland white bread makes the perfect foil for flavourful toppings, cheeses and cured meats. Rarely is stale bread thrown out; instead, it is added to soups and stews to soak up the juices.

I am not a baker, but I was recently invited to a bread-baking party. Similar to the pasta-making classes we hold at the villa, these get-togethers have the warm feel of a good book club, only with aprons! The bread that came out of the oven at the end was lovely, but the true wonder was the people mixing and kneading together as the conversation reached new heights of delightful silliness.

Grains and Rice

Beyond the everyday Italian cuisine of bread, pasta and pizza, there are numerous varieties of healthy whole grains used in what was once known as *cucina povera*, the traditional meatless recipes of the poor. As previously mentioned, the industrial-ization and refining of modern grain crops gives them a higher glycemic index; as a result, people often find them inflammatory and hard to tolerate, and thus avoid them. But in their place many highly nutritious ancient grains have been reintro-duced and are now readily available. These grains have become a staple for vege-tarians and vegans, but everyone will enjoy their flavour and health benefits.

My favourite dish on the menu of the mom-and-pop-style restaurant near us is a steaming bowl of Italian wild rice mixed with spelt and steamed asparagus heads, sau-téed mushrooms, lemon juice, a splash of olive oil and salt and pepper—I am drooling just thinking about it. But the waiter there fancies himself quite the comedian. Every time I order it, he grins and says to the entire table, "*Questo ti manterrà regolare*," which you have probably guessed means "This will keep you regular." Embarrassing, but so true.

As Jacky says, roughage is imperative for a healthy, well-functioning digestive tract. It's easy to get enough of it if you replace most of the refined grains in your diet with whole-grain wheat, brown and black rice, farro, spelt, emmer, oats, barley, buckwheat and quinoa. Yup, they will keep you *regolare*.

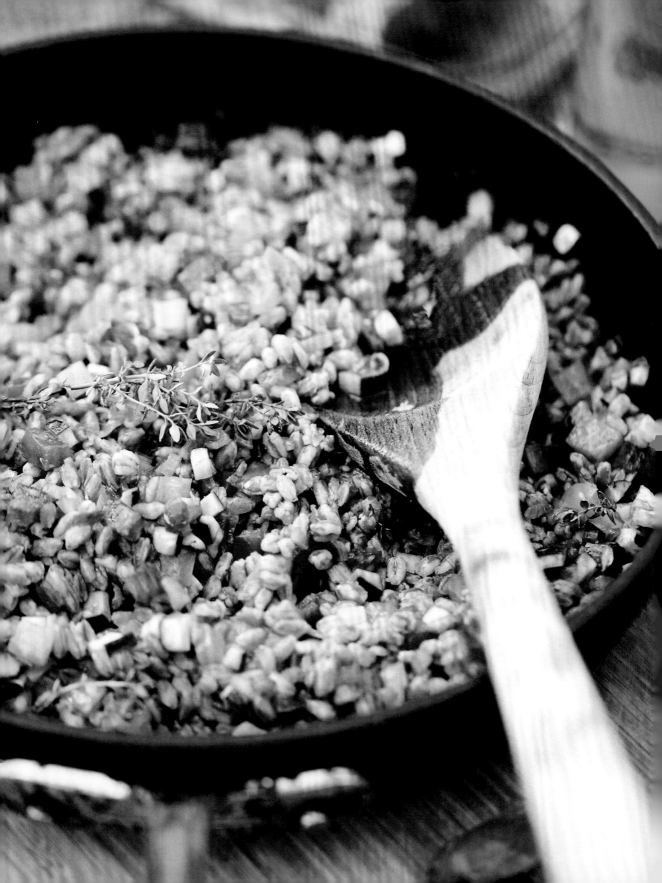

FARRO SALAD WITH BASIL PESTO

SERVES 8

Farro is an ancient crop—it's even mentioned in the Old Testament. This yummy, chewy grain is a mainstay at the villa in soups and salads or as a substitute in rice-based dishes. Flour ground from farro makes for a nutty-tasting bread that is higher in protein and lower in gluten than wheat flour bread and is also a high source of fibre.

We serve this whole-grain farro salad to our guests for a poolside lunch, and any leftovers are even tastier the next day. If you're making it for yourself, a batch cooked on a Sunday will carry you through half the week. Scoop it into large radicchio or iceberg lettuce leaves for a snack, or add a little stock to make a soup—it's always ready when you are.

BASIL PESTO:

½ cup pine nuts

2 cloves garlic, peeled and smashed with flat side of a knife

4 cups fresh basil leaves

½ cup extra virgin olive oil

Salt and freshly ground pepper (to taste, from a pinch each to as much as a teaspoon)

½ cup freshly grated Parmesan cheese

FARRO SALAD:

3 cups dry farro

3 tablespoons extra virgin olive oil

1 yellow bell pepper, finely diced

1 red bell pepper, finely diced

1 red onion, finely diced

1 zucchini, finely diced

1 cup roughly chopped fresh parsley

Salt and freshly ground pepper

To make the pesto: In a small frying pan, over medium heat, lightly toast the pine nuts for 2 minutes, stirring constantly.

Add the garlic, basil, olive oil, salt and pepper to a food processor fitted with a steel blade. Toss in the toasted pine nuts and process until combined. Spoon the mixture into a bowl and gently stir in the Parmesan cheese. Set aside.

To make the farro salad: In large pot, combine the farro and 9 cups of water. Bring to a boil over high heat, then lower the heat and simmer, uncovered, for 25 to 30 minutes or until the farro is chewy but firm (or cook farro according to the package instructions). Drain and set aside.

Meanwhile, in a large frying pan, heat the oil over medium-high heat. Sauté the yellow pepper, red pepper, red onion and zucchini for 5 minutes, until softened.

In a large serving bowl, mix together the farro, vegetable mixture and parsley. Season to taste with salt and pepper. Serve warm or at room temperature. The pesto can either be mixed into the salad or offered in a separate dish so everyone can add their own hearty dollop on top.

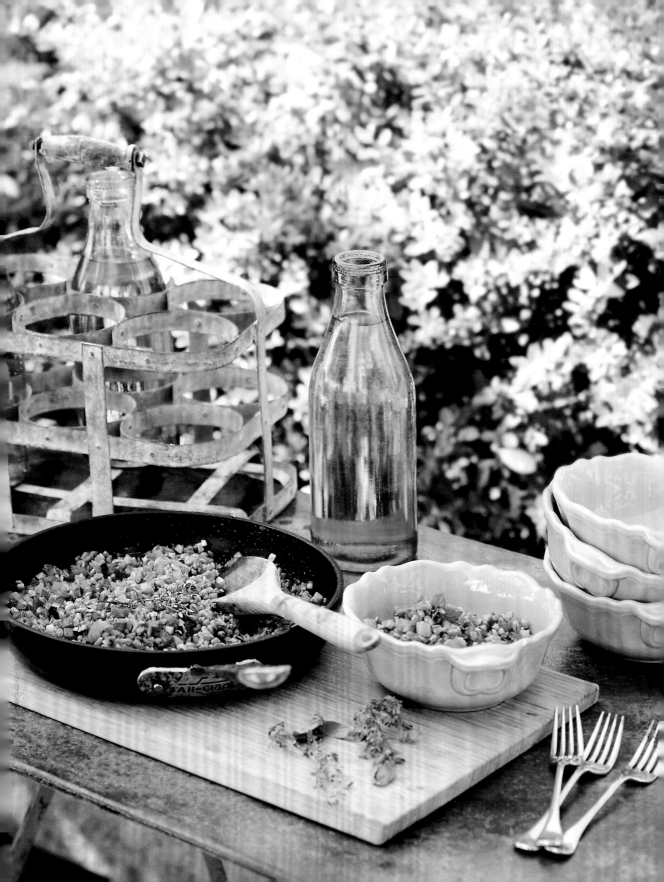

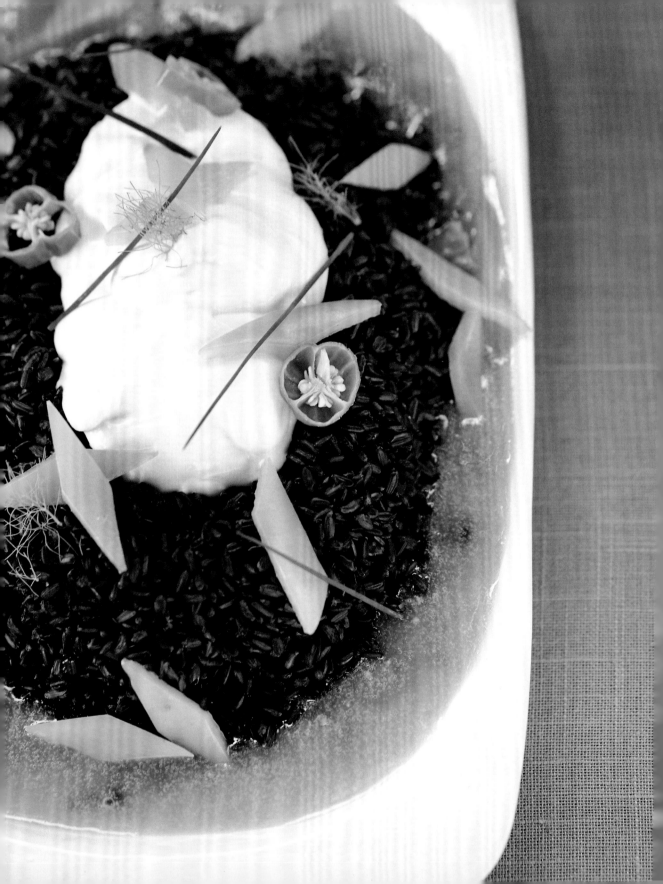

BLACK RISOTTO

Whenever we serve Chef Francesco's glossy, steaming black risotto, a reverential silence reigns as the guests begin to eat. Inevitably, the spell is broken by someone loudly announcing, "This is the most awesome thing I've ever tasted!" There is heavy competition for primacy amongst the varieties of this classic Italian dish, but Chef's version could certainly win medals.

Every region, village, household and cook has their own carefully guarded risotto recipe. Some are creamy and rich, with mushrooms or peas or a handful of shellfish thrown in; spring versions are topped with wild nettles or peas. In the Chianti region, the rice is cooked in red wine. Risotto is made with plump short-grain rice, most commonly arborio, which releases starch during the cooking, giving the dish its velvety texture. It is usually served as a *prima* (first course), with a portion size of just 1 cup. If enjoyed as a full meal, it is accompanied by a crisp leafy salad or spring vegetables.

Chef Francesco's intense and fragrant risotto may be eaten hot or cold all year round.

BLACK RICE:

2 onions, sliced

3 pinches of salt

2 cups black rice
(such as riso integrale nero
or riso nerone integrale)

YELLOW CARAMEL:

2 yellow bell peppers, cut in half
and seeds removed

¼ cup granulated sugar

3 tablespoons extra virgin olive oil

Two pinches of salt

CHEESE GANACHE:

½ cup coarsely grated aged
pecorino or Grana Padano cheese

½ cup whipping (heavy) cream

SAUTÉED ONIONS:

2 tablespoons extra virgin olive oil

2 large onions, finely diced

Splash of Tuscan dessert wine
(Vin Santo), ice wine or sherry
(or red wine if you prefer less
sweetness)

TO SERVE:

Fennel fronds

Chopped fresh chives

Very thinly sliced sweet chili peppers
(such as friggitelli or cubanelle)

For the rice: Add 5 cups of cold water, the sliced onions and the salt to a large pot and bring to a boil over high heat. Lower the heat and simmer for 1 hour. Using a large slotted spoon, remove and discard the onions.

Bring the clear broth in the pot to a boil over high heat. Add the rice, lower the heat and simmer for 25 minutes, until tender. Drain in a fine-mesh strainer.

To make the yellow caramel: Set a medium pot of water over high heat. Bring to a boil and add the yellow peppers and cook for 5 minutes. Drain and let cool, then remove stems and seeds.

In a small pot, combine the sugar and 1 cup of water. Cook over low heat for 10 minutes, stirring occasionally, until the sugar has dissolved, creating a simple syrup.

Slice the cooled peppers into ½-inch (1 cm) thick strips. Reserve half of the strips for garnish. Add the remaining strips to a food processor fitted with a steel blade, along with the simple syrup, olive oil and salt. Process into a smooth, thick liquid. Set aside.

For the ganache: In a glass or metal heatproof bowl, combine the pecorino and cream. Fill a small pot half full with water and bring to a low boil over medium heat. Place the heatproof bowl on top of the pot, making sure the bottom does not touch the boiling water, and cook for 10 minutes, stirring frequently. Place the bowl in the fridge to cool for 15 minutes. Once cool, whisk for a couple of minutes, until thick.

For the onions: Meanwhile, in a large frying pan, heat the olive oil over medium-low heat. Add the diced onions and sauté for about 10 minutes, until lightly browned. Add a splash of wine, increase the heat to medium-high and sauté for about 1 minute.

To serve: Whether you're serving the risotto in individual portions or family-style on a big platter, start by arranging the sautéed onions as the base of your dish. Next, add the black rice on top and evenly pour the yellow caramel around the rice. Add the ganache in a dollop on top and garnish all over with fennel fronds, chives, chili peppers and the reserved yellow pepper strips.

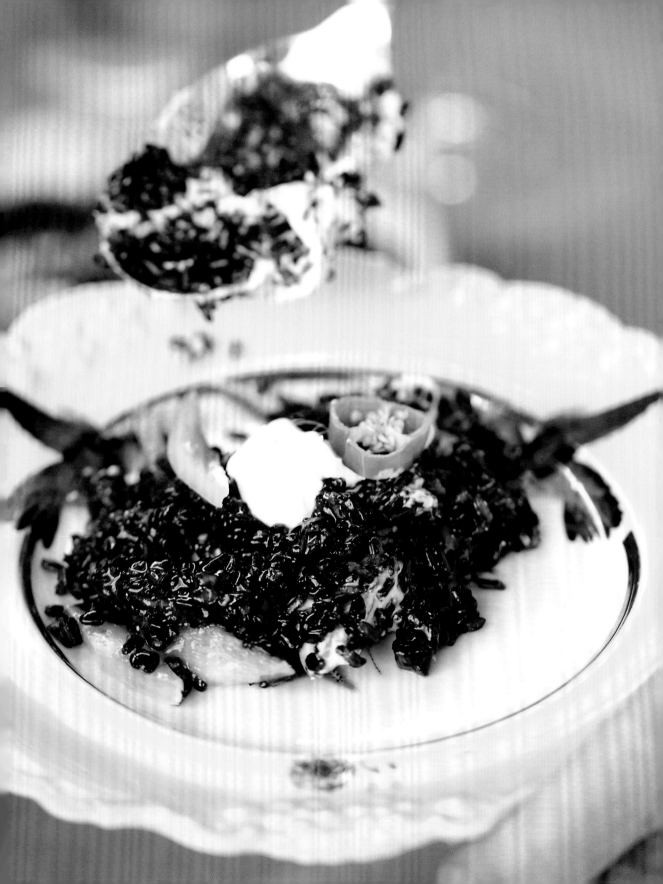

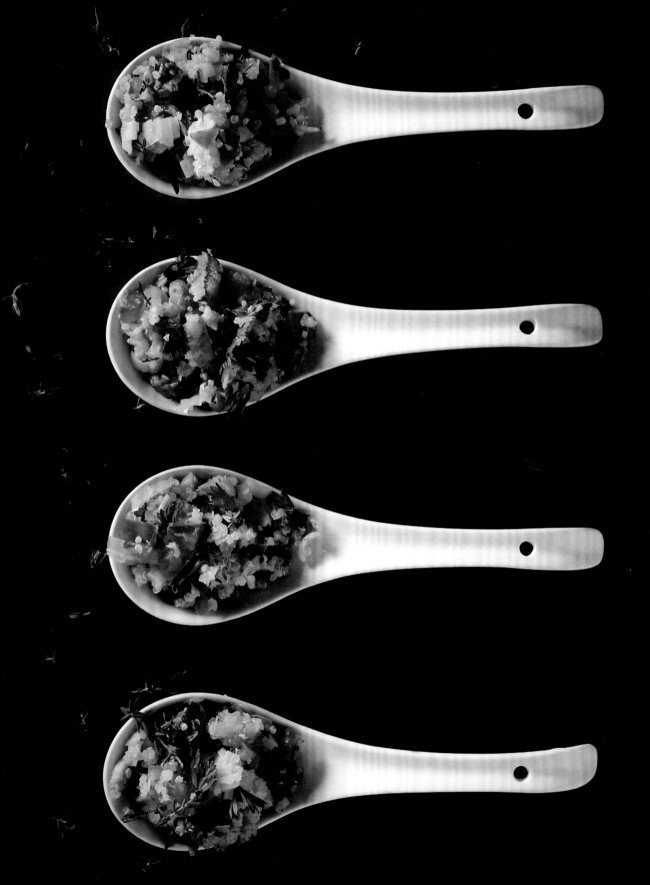

CHEF FRANCESCO'S
SPECIAL QUINOA PANZANELLA

SERVES 6 TO 8

The traditional panzanella, a salad popular for hot summer lunches, is not my favourite, and I always felt guilty that I seemed to be the only person who did not ooh and ahh over this dish. Then Chef Francesco invented his own version—I like to think just for me. Panzanella is peasant food, taking leftover bread and livening it up with summer tomatoes and olive oil. For his version, Chef swaps quinoa for the bread, making the salad both tastier and highly nutritious. It's an ideal substitute for anyone avoiding gluten, and is also a good source of protein. We serve it either as a side dish or on decorative spoons during an *aperitivo*.

4 tablespoons extra virgin olive oil

2 large leeks, white parts only, finely chopped (about 2 cups)

1 clove garlic, minced

½ cup sweet wine (Vin Santo or ice wine)

2 cups very finely chopped tomatoes

3 big pinches of salt

2 cups quinoa, rinsed

1 tablespoon chopped fresh thyme (or 1 teaspoon dried)

1 tablespoon chopped fresh parsley

Freshly ground pepper

In a large frying pan, heat the olive oil over medium heat. Sauté the leeks and garlic for a few minutes, until soft and translucent. Add the wine and cook for 1 minute to allow some of the alcohol to evaporate. Add the tomatoes and salt, lower the heat and simmer gently for about 20 minutes, until the tomatoes are soft.

Meanwhile, in a medium pot bring 4 cups of salted water to a boil over high heat. Add the quinoa, lower the heat and simmer for 15 to 20 minutes or until the water is absorbed and the quinoa is tender.

Stir the quinoa into the leek mixture, along with the thyme and parsley. Season to taste with pepper.

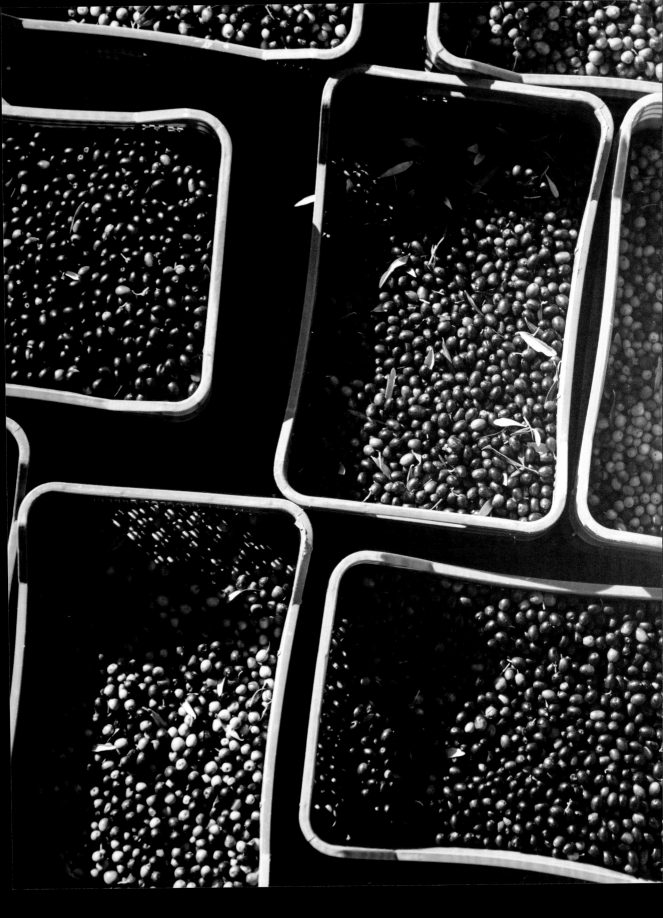

The Wild World of Olive Oil

When I was a little girl, the only olive oil I knew about was medicinal. My mum would buy a tiny bottle from the pharmacy, warm the liquid and then pour it gently into my ears to unblock them. Never would she envision tossing the stuff onto a salad. "Foreign food"—which was anything other than our standard British nosh—was not part of our diets. The inhabitants of Mediterranean and Middle Eastern countries have been well aware of the benefits of extra virgin olive oil for thousands of years, but it took until relatively recently for word to get out to the rest of us.

I'm sure my mother wouldn't know what to make of the fact that her daughter now takes care of a hundred acres of olive trees. By mid-October the landscape is strewn with giant nets ready to catch the olives, a truly special fruit. Hillsides are cluttered with families, friends and workers combing, picking and shaking the plump ripe olives from the trees. It is the most magical time of year.

Our first harvest took place before the renovation of the buildings had begun. "Those trees won't pick themselves!" Luciano, the farmer we'd inherited with the property, proclaimed to us newcomers as we stared aghast at the sea of swaying trees, over fifteen hundred of them. Surrounded by our sons and every Tom, Dick and Giovanni we could muster, we picked throughout the day until the sun sank over the far-off cluster of cypress trees. We carted heavy crates overflowing with black, green and blood-red olives to the local *frantoia*, where we stood amongst our farming neighbours to witness the first press. It was an experience that felt to me as intense as any religious ceremony—an affirmation of the bounty gifted us by the land. Each day we saluted our hard work by celebrating with picnics of bread toasted on a bonfire, rubbed with garlic and rough salt and finally drizzled with the rich green nectar of our own piquant extra virgin olive oil. Five defining weeks: if we'd had any doubts about our decision to move to a remote hillside in Tuscany, they were swept away. The proof that this was our "happy place" was painted across our rapturous faces.

One of my favourite workshops of our retreats is when I gather the guests in the serenity of the olive groves for a chat about how extra virgin olive oil can revolutionize our health. Including olive oil—mostly a monounsaturated fat, with 14 percent saturated fat, and small amounts of vitamins E and K—in our diets is linked to a lower risk of obesity, inflammation, stroke, heart disease, high cholesterol and high blood pressure. The oil's vital fatty acids also assist in the absorption of important vitamins. But we have to learn to be discerning consumers, as commercial olive oil is not all it claims to be.

Worldwide demand for extra virgin olive oil has increased rapidly, and it is predicted to be an $11 billion industry by 2025. But where there are vast profits, corruption rears its ugly head: the adulterating and misrepresentation of olive oil is highly lucrative for unscrupulous players. As Tom Mueller memorably puts it in his book *Extra Virginity: The Sublime and Scandalous World of Olive Oil*, "profits [from fake olive oil] are comparable to cocaine trafficking, with none of the risks."

Just as we decipher the food labels on the back of the bottle, we must also study the front. For olive oil that claims to be Tuscan, if the words "product of Tuscany" don't appear on the label, it is only packaged and bottled in the region and not made from Tuscan olives.

So what is actually in that bottle that's only claiming to be Tuscan? At best, you'll find a blend of oils from olives harvested and pressed in a variety of countries, similar to cheap wine. At worst, it might not be oil extracted from the juice of olives at all, but an inferior oil that has been dyed and flavoured to emulate quality olive oil. I find it heartbreaking to think of someone who has made the decision to ditch processed vegetable oils from their diet and unknowingly buys this stuff, assuming they are now eating a healthier option.

The good news is that there *are* plenty of authentic olive oils readily available. They come from countries such as Spain (the largest producer), Turkey, Greece, Italy (I will always say Tuscan olive oil is the very best, but I am biased), France, Portugal, Australia, California and even a relatively new farming venture in British Columbia, Canada.

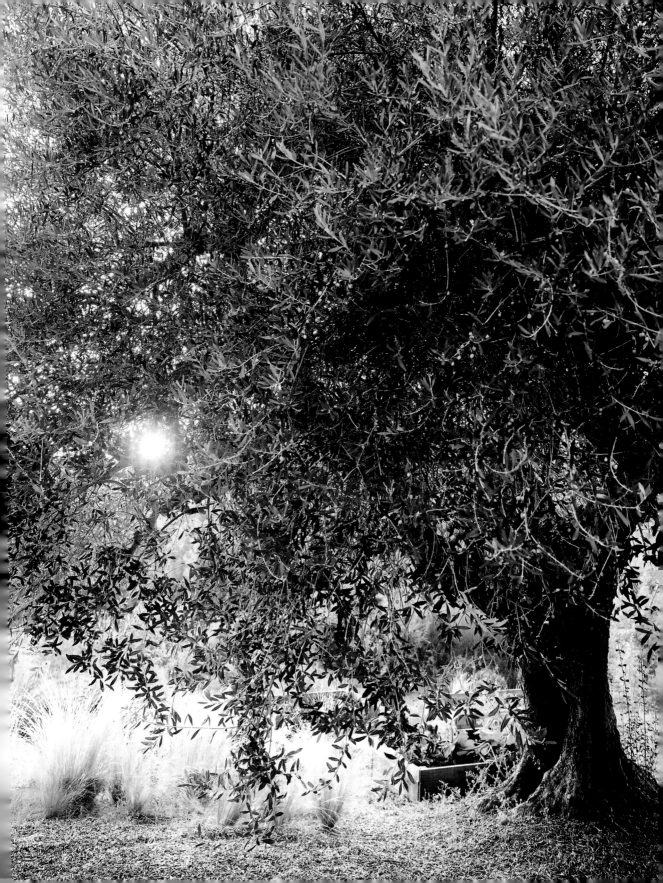

OLIVE OIL IN ALL ITS VARIETIES

Read the Label Carefully!

EXTRA VIRGIN OLIVE OIL: Within hours after being picked by hand, the olives are taken to the mill to be pressed. Extra virgin olive oil is the result of this first pressing. Containing nothing but olives and sunshine, the oil's colour can range from golden to forest green. The flavour is the stuff of legend—spicy and aromatic, evoking romantic visions of an unspoiled landscape. Each batch varies in taste depending on what grows in the earth around the trees. Olive oil from our farm can have hints of wild garlic, asparagus and oregano. (Commercial olive oil is usually an industrialized blend with a consistent flavour.) Make sure the label on the bottle says where the oil is produced. Even better, look for one that names the actual estate.

VIRGIN OLIVE OIL: The mulch from the first press is scooped up into containers and taken to a commercial outlet, where the remaining juice is extracted by chemical process. Virgin olive oil is a lower grade than extra virgin, and the nutritional benefits are lessened, as are the taste, aroma and quality.

REGULAR REFINED OLIVE OIL: Low-end olive oils are blended and heat-refined to remove any unwanted flavours or odours. The oil becomes bland and insipid, and there is a further decline in the health benefits of the product.

PURE OLIVE OIL: Don't be fooled by that tender word *pure*. After being refined by chemical processes, less than 10 percent extra virgin olive oil remains in this product. It is flavourless and has little of the goodness left.

LIGHT OLIVE OIL: Now my blood really begins to boil. There is no one on the planet who reads the word *light* and does not decode it as meaning that a product has fewer calories than one without that designation. But the fat content and calories are the same here: oil is oil. There are approximately 120 calories per tablespoon in whatever edible oil you choose, including light olive oil. The word just means that the refining process makes this oil pale in colour and that the olive flavour is reduced to almost nil.

Bakers often tell me they don't like the pronounced flavour of quality olive oil in their goods, which is why they opt to use light olive oil. In that case, as a healthier alternative, I suggest they should try almond, avocado or coconut oil.

COLD-PRESSED OLIVE OIL: Cold-pressing is a process used to extract the juice from the fruit, similar to squeezing an orange. In the old days, the olives were put on a circular stone plate and a second plate was placed on top to laboriously crush the olives and wring out their nectar. In the modern world, extra virgin olive oil is obtained by cold-pressing the olives with steel plates, using minimal heat, a process that retains the oil's rich scent and flavour, and all of its nutritional goodness.

Refined oils are made by extracting the juice in a process involving high heat and chemicals, reducing the wonderful benefits gained from cold-pressed oil.

ORGANIC OLIVE OIL: Olive trees can be extremely long-lived and hardy, but they are still susceptible to pests, especially the dreaded fruit fly, which destroys the olives. Our farm is organic, which means we never spray with chemical pesticides. Spraying the trees can easily leave a residue of the chemicals on the olives, some of which would make it into the bottle. So we pray for a deep cold spell in late winter to kill off the larva of this pest. If that doesn't happen, we will have to discard the picking, and there will be zero oil for the coming year. It's one of the reasons why organic oil costs more.

Tips for Buying and Keeping the Best Extra Virgin Olive Oil

Extra virgin olive oil is best used within a year, because the nutritional value, flavour and aroma deteriorate over time. Check the expiry or sell-by date on the bottle or can. It is best to find a brand that displays the *harvest* date, which is the best measure of the actual age of the oil when you purchase it.

Until I became fascinated with the world of healthy oil, I bought mine in giant clear plastic containers from discount stores and set them on my kitchen counter. Wrong, wrong and wrong, Debbie. First, if you're not actually going to use huge containers of oil, purchase the quantity that's right for you and your household. Oils do not keep well in clear plastic containers, as the increased oxidation causes the quality to deteriorate. Extra virgin olive oil is at its very best in dark glass bottles or tins. You don't need to store it in the fridge, but keep it out of direct sunlight.

Extra virgin oil is more expensive than the others on offer. But if you think about it, what is the point of using olive oil with inferior goodness and benefits? Oil connoisseurs will tell you that, similar to wines, each extra virgin olive oil has its own specific qualities: some are better for cooking, others for trickling on vegetables, salads and soups. A note of caution: super-expensive oils from fancy gourmet shops can take longer to sell, due to their cost, so remember to check the all-important harvest date. There is nothing worse than rancid oil, especially if you have spent a small fortune on it!

Seek out your local Italian, Portuguese, Greek or Turkish specialty shops; if they know their merchandise, they will be able to guide you toward finding the real deal. Consortiums put together by a group of small farms are another option—they sell in quantity to merchants, but also facilitate direct online ordering by individuals; in fact, that's how we sell our oil. We have a limited batch each year, about two thousand bottles, and after reserving five hundred or so for family and to serve at the villa, we sell the rest online. When you order this way, you know exactly where the oil is from. Many individual olive farms and small hotels around southern Europe take part in this venture: they grow the olives and harvest, press and ship the oil to you directly. What a wonderful way to buy this healthy staple.

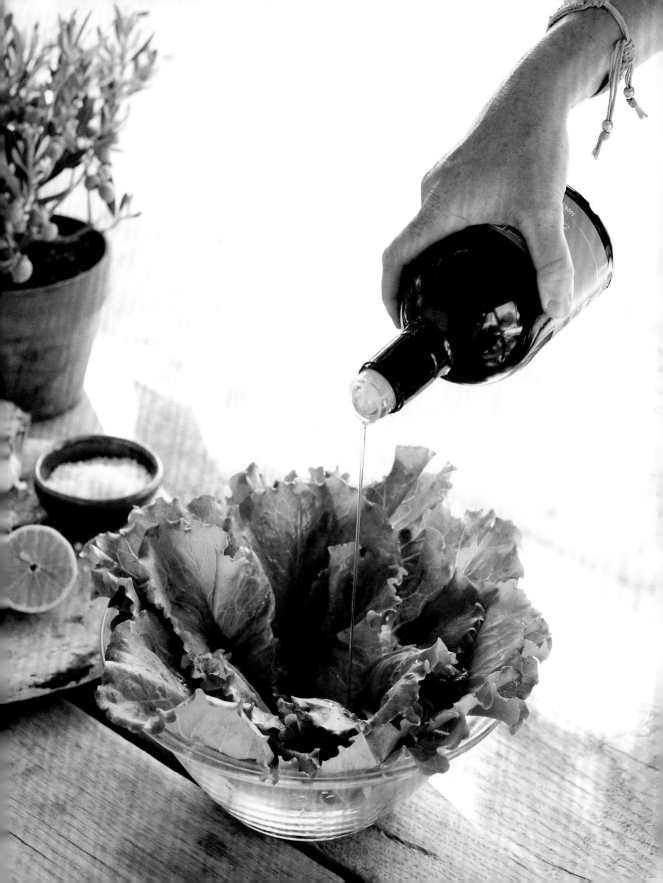

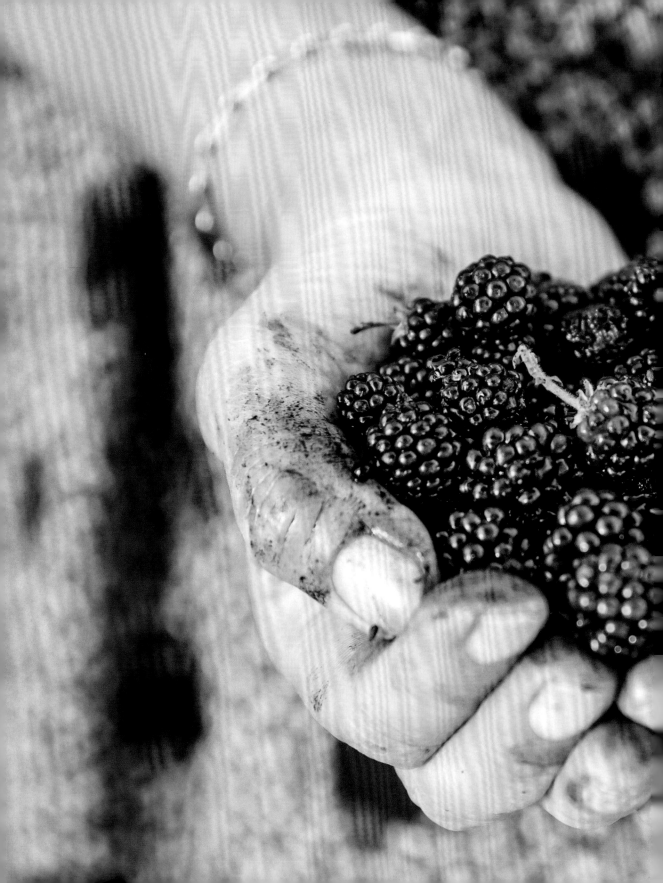

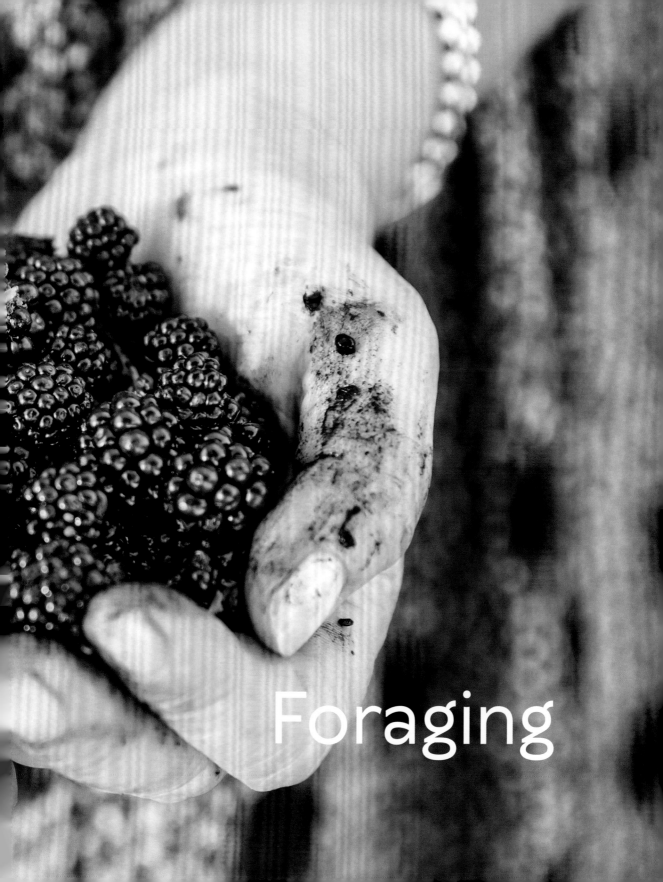

Foraging

the side of Tuscan dirt roads, backs bent, knee-deep in the undergrowth, foraging for wild greens, berries and herbs. So we think it's only fitting that we schedule a foraging morning during our retreats. Rising at dawn, we head into the woods like sleepy soldiers, marching on ground that's still heavy with dew. The group is always bemused at first, wondering if I have gone a bit mad. But it never fails: we return enlivened, carrying baskets of knowledge and wild mushrooms, mint, oregano, skinny stalks of asparagus, miniature bulbs of garlic, flowering fennel . . . oh, the list is endless.

The foraging mornings are so popular with the guests, everyone wants to join a foraging group back home. Happily, the practice is cropping up like weeds every-where, as groups of city folk throw on rubber boots and head to parks, wasteland and the countryside. It is a brilliant way to get outside and meet up with friends old and new, and is a small but important way to reduce your carbon footprint, thereby helping the environment. Trying new tastes and gathering wild foods is good for your health, and even doing research on the edible herbs and plants common in your area is fun and eye-opening. Let the treasure hunt begin!

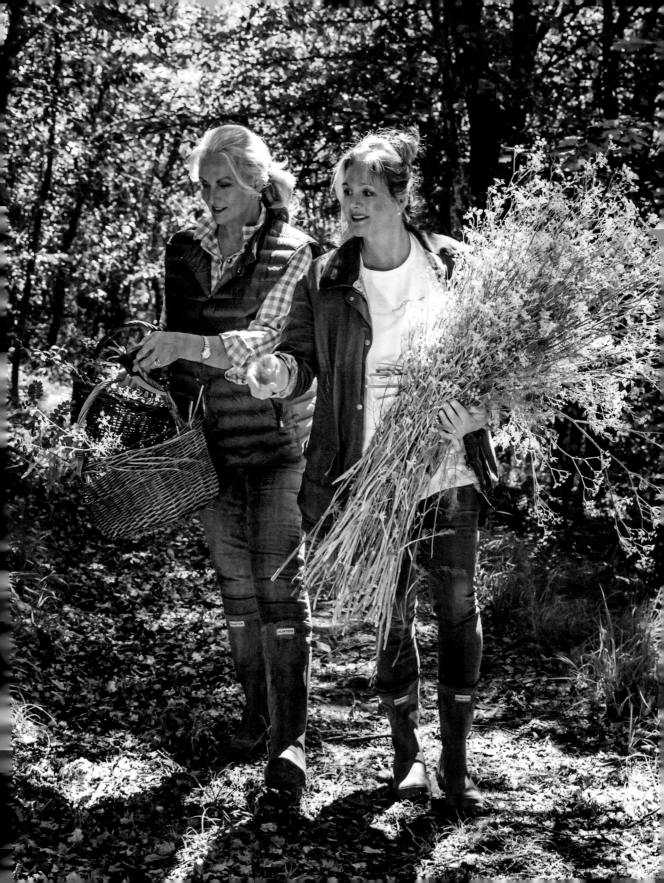

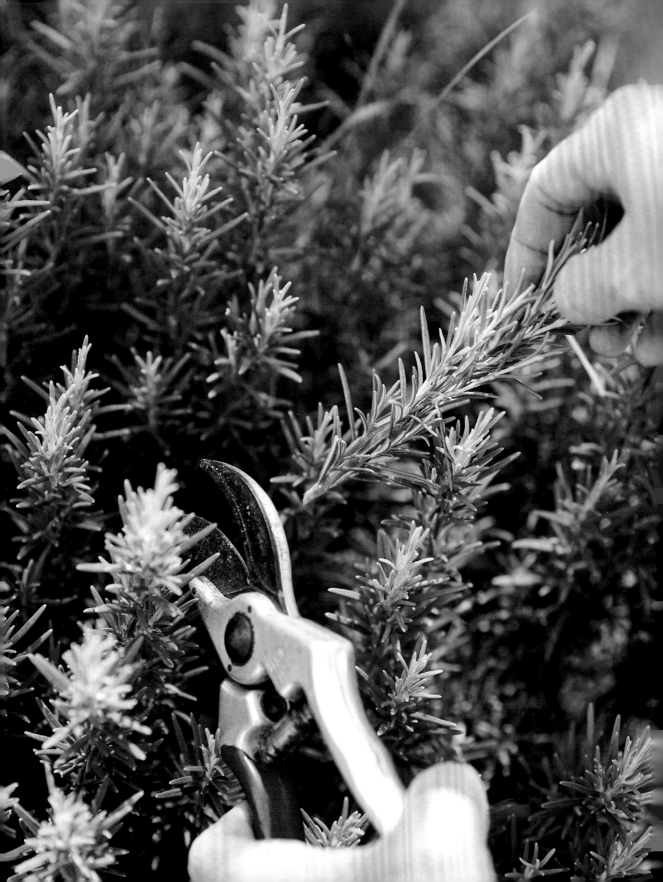

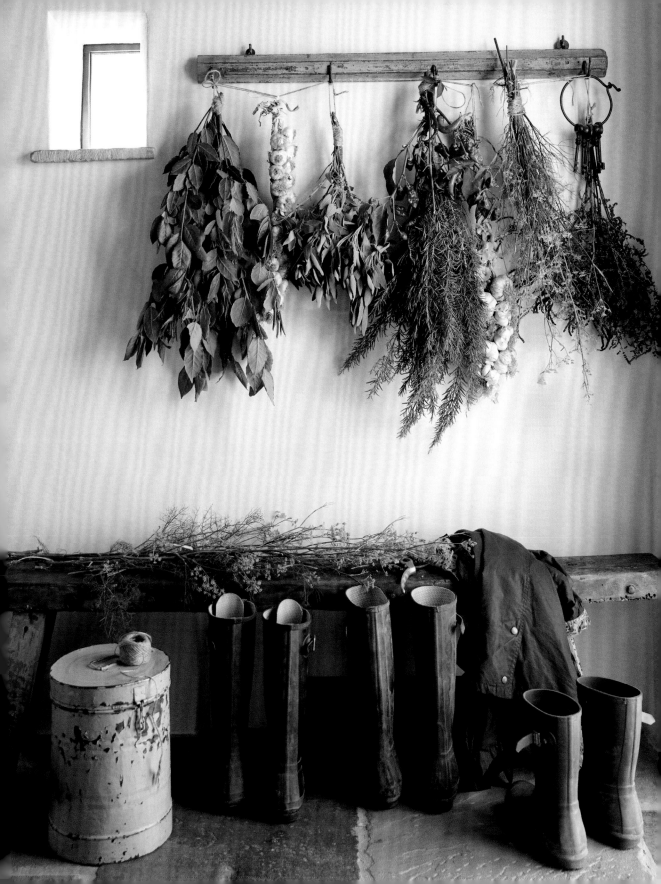

THE BENEFITS OF EVERYDAY HERBS

Herbs are a central component of cooking in all cultures, valued not just for their flavour but also for their medicinal properties. Here at the villa, we find local herbs by foraging in fields and along roadsides, we grow more in pots around the house, and we buy big bunches at farmers' markets and from stores everywhere. Here are some herbs that Italians use faithfully.

OREGANO: sprinkled on grilled vegetables and into stews, is not only packed with flavour, but is both an antioxidant and an anti-inflammatory. The essential oil derived from the plant is also antimicrobial and is now being used in cleaning products in hospitals to fight the superbug methicillin-resistant staphylococcus aureus (MRSA). You can also use the essential oil topically, to treat skin conditions such as fungal infections and acne.

BASIL: is the taste of Italy and can transform a simple sauce into a memorable one. You can reap the health benefits of basil by infusing the dried or fresh leaves in a tea, scattering the fresh leaves over salads and other dishes, or whizzing the fresh leaves into pesto. The flavonoids found in basil fight free radicals, and the essential oil is thought to be protective against inflammation. Jacky says it is an adaptogenic herb—it helps balance the body and fight stress.

GARLIC: is a bulb that is used like a herb. It adds flavour to dishes from many cuisines, but especially Italian cooking. Its medicinal uses date back thousands of years to Central Asia and Northern Iran. What makes garlic so healthy are the sulphur compounds allicin and alliin, which are activated by crushing and chopping. Garlic has antithrombotic effects (it reduces the formation of blood clots), supports the immune system and can be used to treat respiratory conditions. Draping your head with a tea towel and breathing in the steam from a glass bowl of hot water infused with a couple of cloves of crushed garlic is a time-honoured home remedy for stuffy noses caused by the common cold.

ROSEMARY: loved for both its fragrance and its flavour, has culinary, medicinal and commercial uses. It is perhaps best known for being sprinkled on roast lamb and potatoes, but rosemary can be added to all kinds of dishes and drinks. The active compounds, plant polyphenols, account for most of rosemary's anti-oxidant and pharmacological activities. The essential oil, extracted from the leaves, is used in many herbal medicines. We use rosemary religiously at the villa, as this Mediterranean herb is often mentioned as an ingredient of the "fountain of youth." It is also known to help treat osteoarthritis pain and enhance brain function, and rosemary oil rubbed into the scalp is said to stimulate hair growth.

SAGE: packs a good dose of minerals and vitamins, and can be used fresh or dried to flavour food. The volatile oils found in sage leaves have numerous benefits, including antimicrobial, anti-inflammatory and neuroprotective properties. Sage infusions reduce bacteria in the mouth, helping to support oral health.

LAVENDER: is well known for its calming properties (see "Perfumed Nights," page 106). It grows madly around our property, releasing wafts of its distinctive fragrance throughout the summer. Researchers have found that the fragrant volatile oil extracted from lavender blossoms has plenty of medicinal uses. As far back as the Middle Ages, these purple flowers were used as a home remedy for stress, hysteria, menopausal symptoms, anxiety, headaches and even convulsions and fainting spells. In more modern times, lavender oil became an important ingredient in smelling salts. Lavender has recently enjoyed a resurgence in popularity and is once again being added to oils, diffusers and creams as an antioxidant, an anti-inflammatory and a sedative, and to treat metabolic disorders.

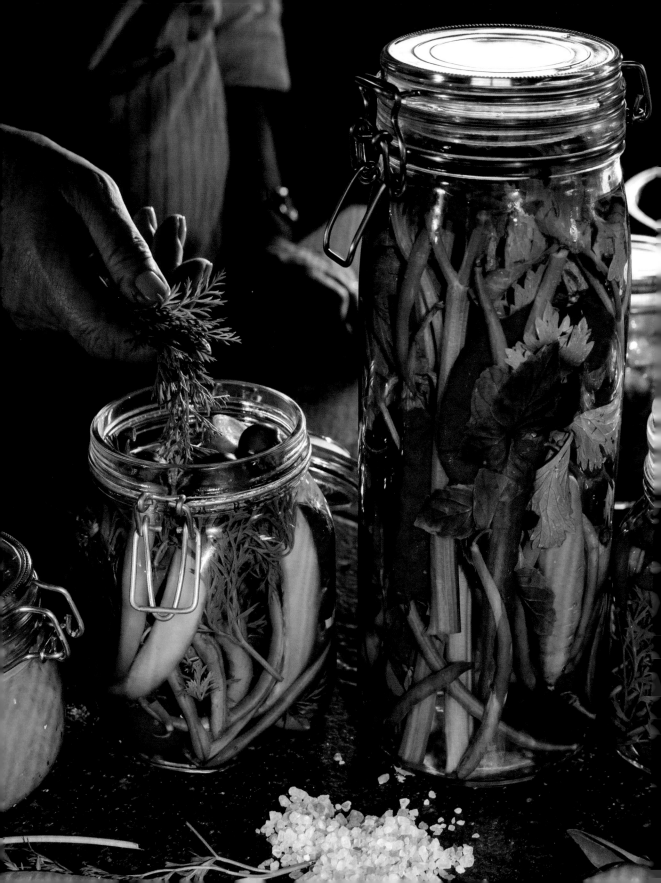

Fermenting

Our fermenting classes always begin with puzzlement about what on earth we are making. But fermented food is actually quite common; in fact, many of our daily foods—cheese, chocolate, wine, beer, yogurt and even bread—are produced by some form of fermentation.

Fermenting is a natural way to preserve food and drink, a process that can be traced back thousands of years. Imagine a world before fridges. The first fermentation is thought to have been mead, a combination of honey and water. The natural yeast in the raw honey activated the fermentation process, producing a delicious and intoxicating liquid. Early humans knew how to have a good time.

All nations have some form of fermented food that goes back centuries, enabling them to store different perishables throughout the year. The Inuit and other Indigenous Peoples in Canada's north have igunaq, fermented walrus, while Germans consume lots of sauerkraut, made from green cabbage. The Japanese ferment soybeans to make pungent, gelatinous natto, a traditional breakfast staple. In Russia and Turkey, shepherds made a fermented milk drink kept in skins and hung over their doorways; as people entered and left the home, the skins would take a knocking, agitating the milk and helping the fermentation process.

However, until about twenty years ago, the art of fermenting at home had been almost forgotten—in North America, particularly. The re-emerging interest in this technique is at least in part a response to research showing that the friendly bacteria fermentation produces can help protect against numerous twenty-first century diseases. Many of us are cottoning on to the appeal of naturally fermented food and trying our hand at fermenting in our own homes rather than relying on commercial preparations, many of which have been pasteurized and are therefore no longer "alive," meaning their benefits are greatly reduced. One note of caution. It's ideal to eat some fermented foods every day, but introduce them slowly, so your digestive system has a chance to become accustomed to them.

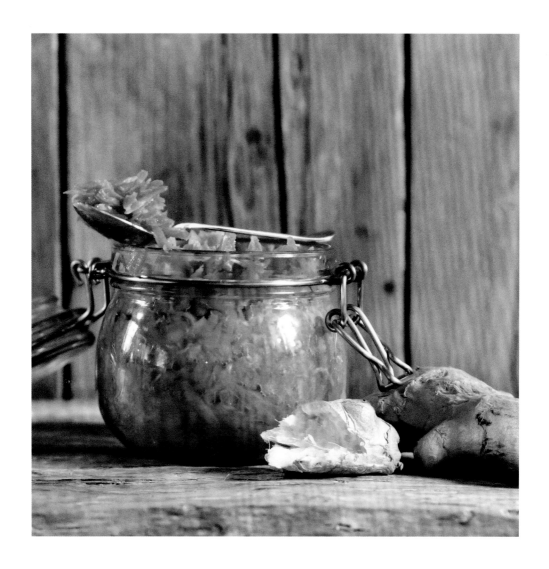

JOY

FERMENTED CARROTS with FRESH GINGER

Here is an easy starter recipe that you can adapt to most other vegetables, too. Peppers, zucchini, garlic, cabbage, cauliflower—whatever you find more appealing or a combo of all! Just apply the same method I describe below.

    1 pound (450 g) organic carrots
    3 tablespoons grated fresh ginger
    1½ teaspoons good sea salt or Himalayan salt
    Filtered water (if needed)

Sterilize a 2-cup (500 ml) Mason jar, lid and ring by washing them in the dishwasher or boiling them in water for 5 minutes. Set aside to air-dry.

After giving the carrots a good scrub, coarsely grate or thinly slice them. In a large bowl, using clean hands, knead the carrots, ginger and salt together until the carrot juices run freely. Let sit for 30 minutes at room temperature.

Pack the carrots firmly into the jar. If the juices don't cover them, top up with a little filtered water until they are submerged, leaving a half-inch of headspace. If necessary, place fermentation weights on top of the carrots to keep them under the liquid. Wipe the jar rim, cover with the lid and screw on the ring until fingertip-tight.

Set the jar in a dark, cool room for at least 3 days or up to 10 days (the carrots will become more fermented and tangier the longer you leave them). Taste each day, and when you achieve the flavour you desire, eat! If you don't get through them in one meal and want to stop the fermentation process, put the jar in the fridge and eat within 3 months.

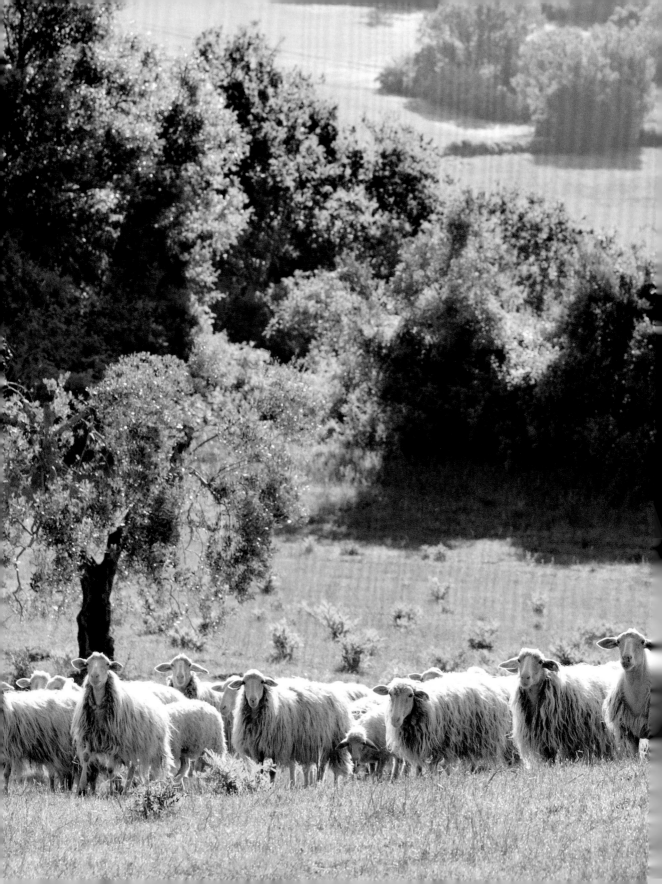

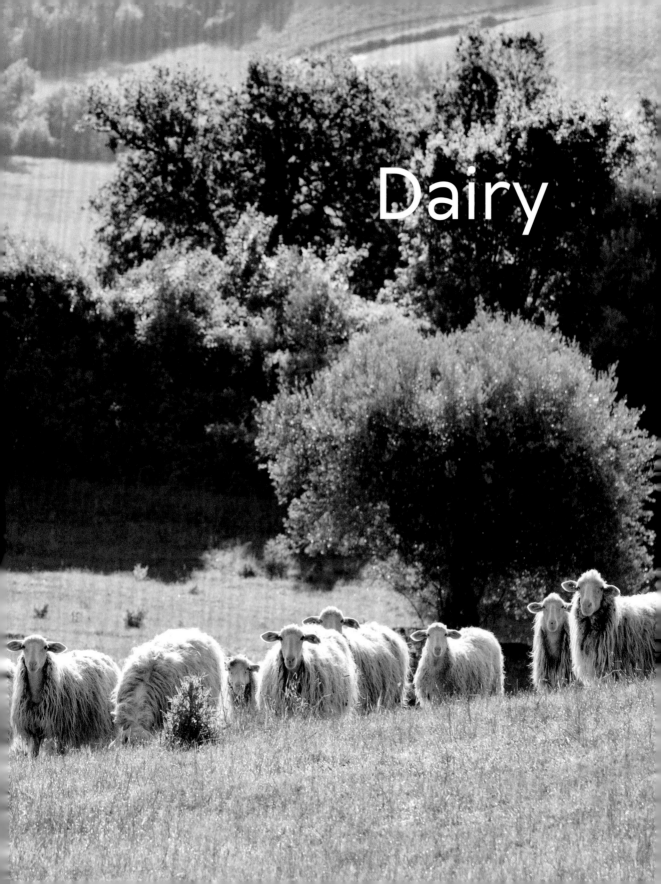

Dairy

DAIRY CONSUMPTION IN ITALY TENDS TO VARY FROM REGION TO REGION. In the north, where the weather is cooler and more rain falls, the green pastures feed herds of dairy cows. In the areas south of Rome, the climate is drier and there are fewer milk products. Despite the abundance of transportation options today, traditions stand firm in this land, especially when it comes to food. While pasta and pizza are staple meals in both the north and the south, the sauces and toppings are completely different. In the south, the dishes are tomato-based; in the north, they are cheese-based—think marinara compared to carbonara. People across the country indulge in gelato (which is usually dairy-based), yet cream is used in only a few desserts, and butter is not a staple in the Italian kitchen.

It may be hard to believe, but most Italians do not eat masses of cheese, and what they do consume is of the highest quality. It is unusual to see mounds of grated cheese added to bowls of spaghetti, as you might see in an American-style Italian restaurant. When they nibble from a cheese board, usually during an *aperitivo*, the portions are sliver-sized and served alongside honey, some nuts and dried fruit, all tantalizing the taste buds together.

Tuscany lies north of Rome, and here the long, hot, dry summers produce a short grass that is loved by sheep. Most of the milk used to make the region's different varieties of cheese come from these sheep, and since the word for "sheep" in Italian is *pecora*, the cheeses are known as pecorino. These are the cheeses we serve at the villa, and even our guests who consider themselves lactose-intolerant often find that they can eat them. There are a couple of reasons why that's the case. First, there are fewer additives in Italian dairy products than in North American dairy products. In addition, all aged cheese has less lactose than fresh because the natural bacteria created during the aging process feeds on lactose, so that after a few months it has nearly all gone. As a result, many people find sheep's milk and goat's milk more easily digestible than cow's milk.

We should all be guided by how the Tuscans enjoy their cheese: small portions of the highest quality, made with few preservatives. Luckily, good-quality imported and locally produced pecorino, made from either sheep's or goat's milk, is widely available in North America and is vastly preferable to the processed

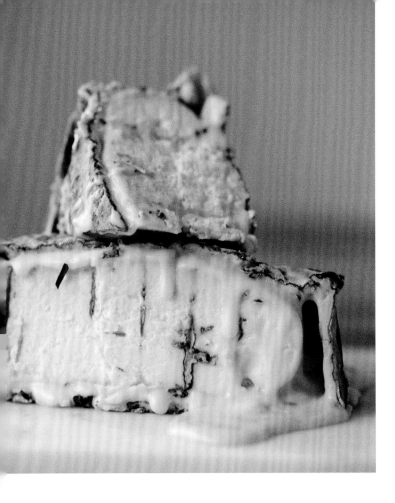

supermarket variety.

When it comes to the trend for alternatives to cow's milk, plant-based non-dairy "cheeses" have landed in Italy just as they have everywhere else. Coconut milk, soy milk, nut milk, hemp milk, oat milk and all the rest are no longer fringe alternatives but compete with cow's milk as a supposedly "better" food choice. But Jacky says to beware—these alternatives can be highly processed, so check labels for thickeners, added sugar and a variety of other additives. Find one you like the taste of and ensure it is as natural as possible. These dairy-free options are a fantastic alternative if you are lactose-intolerant or wish to consume less dairy, as long as you know what to look for.

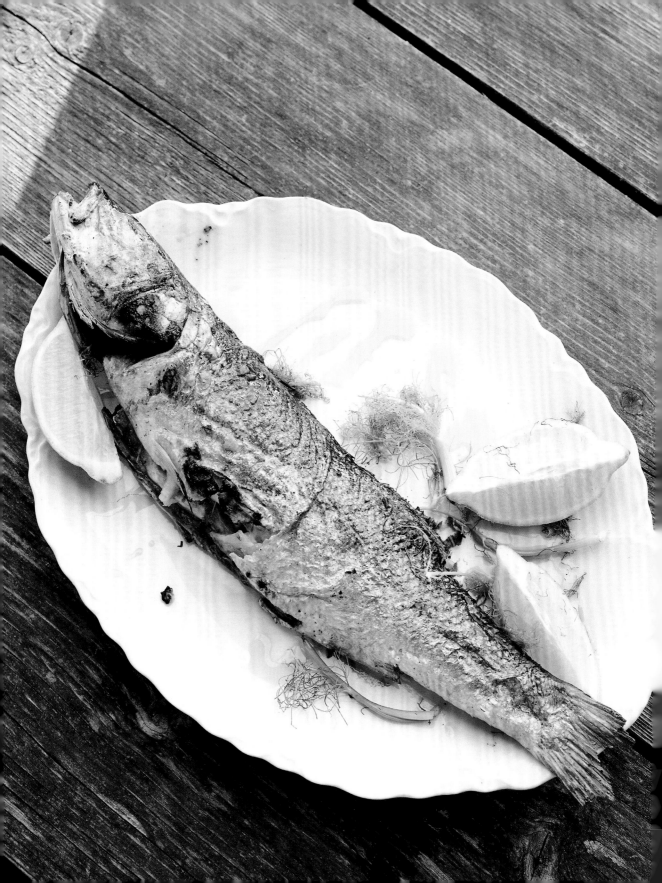

Meat and Fish

The way the Tuscans eat meat and fish is a reminder to us all that less is more.

When I was growing up in England, "posh" meat was a treat—a Sunday roast shared around a noisy table at a family get-together. Meals during the rest of the week relied on whatever meat was on special at the butchers, stretched in the most innovative ways. My mother was a wiz at feeding a large family on a budget. She could produce a shepherd's pie with only a handful of ground meat, packing it with onions, peas and lentils so that it was still completely satisfying. You could barely spot the carne in her chili con carne, it was so full of kidney beans. The classic stew in the North of England is Lancashire hotpot, made from lamb and thinly sliced potatoes and carrots. For her version, my mum used what we called "scrag-end," the fleshy part of the sheep's neck. It sounds dreadful, but it was mouth-watering, inexpensive and highly nutritious.

I was in my late teens before I saw an entire grilled fish, head and tail included. My family ate scraps of fish baked into a pie, or a boil-in-a-bag lump of haddock slathered in a slimy parsley sauce (the horror). If we were really lucky, Mum brought home fish and chips on a Friday night. Back then, it was often cod, since before overfishing that was the cheapest fish, and it was deep-fried in thick batter and served with fat chips splattered in malt vinegar, all of which we inhaled out of folded newspapers. Hardly sophisticated, but oh, what a treat.

We now know that eating small amounts of meat and fish alongside plenty of plant-based foods is a very healthy approach. Following such a diet benefits not only our bodies, but also the environment. If you are fond of meat and all the sea's bounty, enjoy them occasionally, in small portions, and always eat the freshest and best-quality options you can find.

The Tuscans have eaten this way for centuries. In a generally impoverished region, meat was scarce and expensive and, just as in the Northern England of my childhood, it was saved for special occasions. For daily protein, Tuscans still rely mostly on beans, but when they are eating in restaurants, they delight in roasted or grilled dishes of pork, beef, chicken, duck or wild boar. At home, if they are

JACKY SAYS

Premium-quality, unprocessed fish and meat are packed full of bioavailable nutrients and provide an excellent source of protein. All of the animal proteins we consume contain the nine essential amino acids the body needs to build proteins and synthesize hormones and neurotransmitters. Amino acids are also vital for muscle growth and repair, and for preventing muscle loss. Protein deficiencies can have a negative impact on our nervous, reproductive, immune and digestive systems.

Iron is needed for healthy blood. While there is a small amount of iron in many foods, including leafy green vegetables, the best source is red meat. Oily fish, such as salmon, mackerel and sardines, are a good source of omega-3 fatty acids, which fight inflammation, amongst a plethora of other health benefits. And shellfish are a good source of zinc.

For optimal health, purchase good-quality pasture-raised meat, wild-caught salmon, ethically produced shellfish and organic produce. They cost more, but keep in mind we don't need as much meat as is often readily consumed.

Vegans get their protein solely from plant sources and must be sure to consume a wide range of legumes, nuts, seeds, whole grains, fermented tofu and tempeh. One of my favourite vegan sources of amino acids is nutritional yeast, which has a nutty, cheesy flavour and can be added to any food or mixed into a smoothie.

There is a great deal of confusion about how much protein is actually in food. For example, a portion of chicken breast weighing 100 grams does not provide 100 grams of protein—it's actually about 31 grams. A good protein checker app will help eliminate guesswork. To calculate your daily protein needs, a good rule of thumb is to multiply your weight in kilograms by 0.8. So if you weigh 60 kilos, you need 48 grams of protein a day.

eating meat, they tend to serve up lower-grade cuts, often stewed with herbs and deliciously tenderized to enhance the flavour. For true extravagance—enjoyed by tourists, yes, but also by Tuscans when there is cause for celebration—people share the famous bistecca alla Fiorentina, a gigantic T-bone seared on an open fire.

You will also find, hanging in barns, cellars and garages across Italy, a variety of home-cured meats—salami, pepperoni and other sausages of all descriptions. Because they could be stored at room temperature for long periods of time, they were there for people when the supply of fresh meat was scanty, eaten thinly sliced in sandwiches and atop pizzas, or adding zing to stews. The fermentation process that results from salting the meat, usually pork, and letting it age at room temperature allows good organisms to grow and prevents the not-so-good ones from spoiling the meat. The Italians flavour these cured meats with fennel seeds, garlic, pepper, vinegar and even wine; each recipe is as unique as the person making it.

Where we live, in the centre of the country, fish is not common, though you can buy it from *il pescivendolo*, the "fish guy," at the weekly market, and you can usually find octopus and snapper on restaurant menus. But Tuscany also has a long coastline, on the Ligurian and Tyrrhenian seas, where seafood rules. I love fish, and friends and I will drive the two hours to the coast to eat at a particular restaurant, La Dogana Capalbio, a summer pop-up from Rome. We park the car alongside hundreds of others, among rolling sand dunes, and follow the crowds to the beach. There we find our table, perched at the edge of the sea. Bottles of chilled rosé are immediately served, followed by scallops grilled on hot embers and plates piled with spaghetti alla vongole—steaming al dente pasta tossed with clams. There is pan-seared snapper drizzled in chili oil, and bowls of razor clams locally caught that morning.

Why don't they regularly ship some of that fresh fish to my part of Tuscany? As I mentioned earlier, before motorized transport and refrigeration, it took days to get from the coast to places like Montefollonico, and the fish would have gone bad on such a journey. Traditions hold fast here, so every year I make the pilgrimage to the coast for my fish feast.

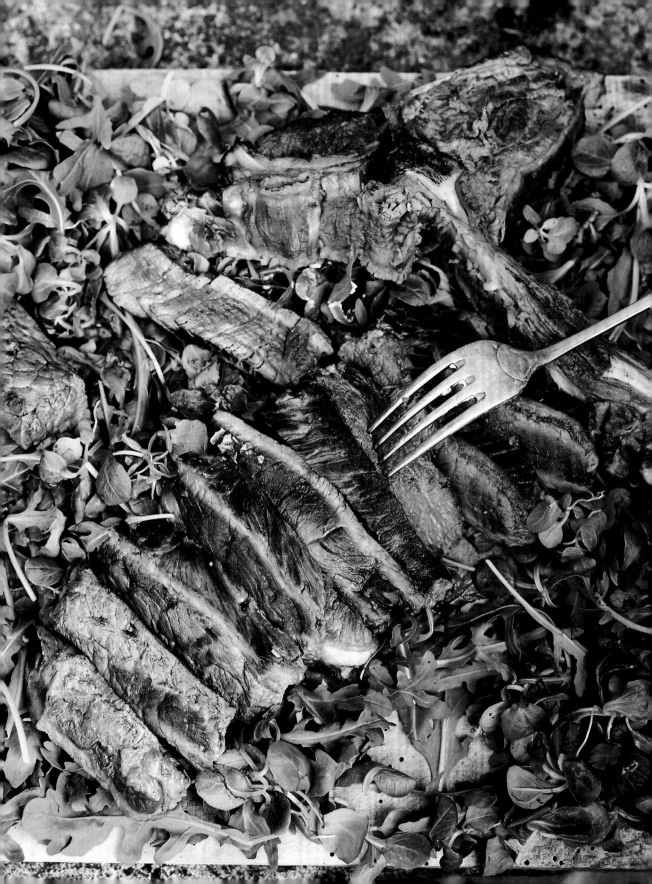

CHEF FRANCESCO

If there is such a person as a true Tuscan, Chef Francesco is it—a man who adores discussing, making and eating Tuscan food. Like so many of his peers, he was raised in a household where everyone lived and breathed for the next meal. "Eating out is a major part of our lifestyle," he says, "but what is much more important to us is 'Mamma's food'—nostalgia, home, hearts and flowers and love, all rolled into one homely meal." It's no wonder he became a chef, when as he says, "I was seduced into cooking for a living by my mother's and grandmother's endless banter about every appetizing delight they were conjuring up." They debated the merits of the last meal and tossed around ideas for the next, even while they were eating the one in front of them into the present one. He laughs when he says, "How can you not be fascinated by the preparation of a dish when it is the constant topic of conversation at home." But when it comes to Tuscan fare, Francesco is quite serious: "For me, the essence of Tuscan cooking is the respect for simple, fresh ingredients, improving on the original and allowing them to shine. I see myself as a wizard who sprinkles a little of this, a little of that and then magic happens. I know this is a worn term, but my happy place is in the kitchen."

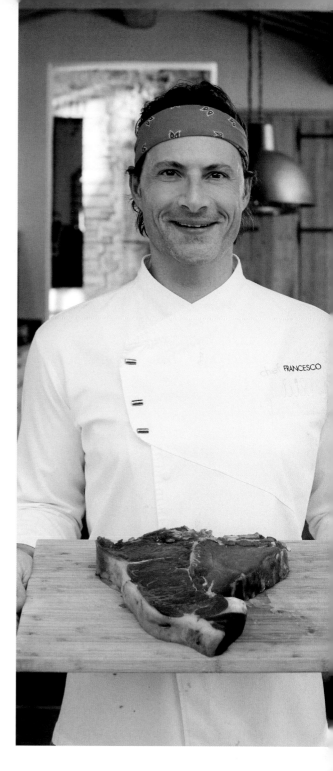

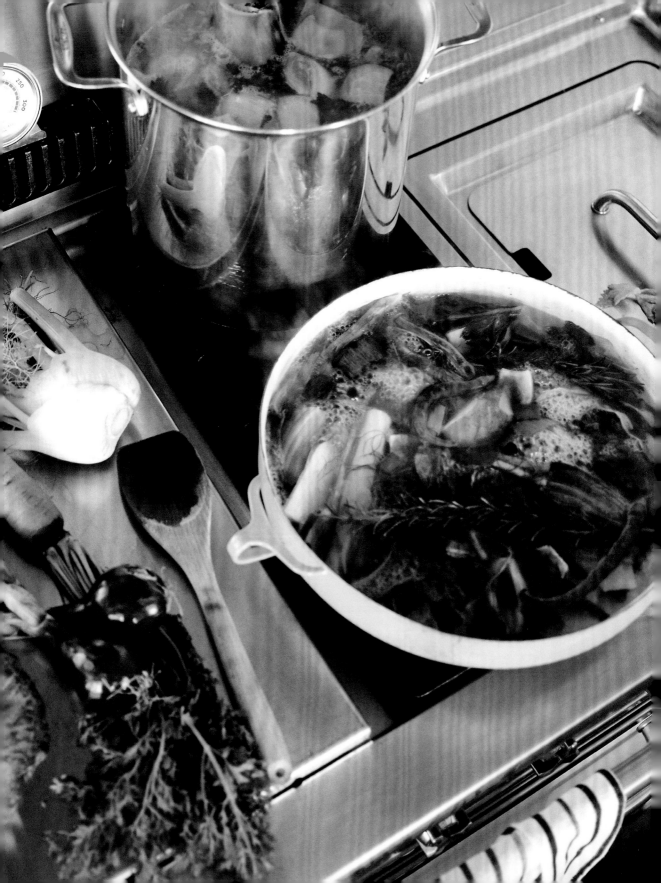

Bone Broth and Vegetable Stock

We have bone broth and vegetable stock on the go throughout the year at the villa, just like every quality restaurant kitchen does. After we've made a large batch, we pour the liquid into portion-sized containers, then freeze. Both of these stocks are easy to make, and incredibly inexpensive.

Bone broth is a protein-dense clear stock that is packed with nutrients due to its lengthy cooking time. It is used as a base for sauces and stews, and is a favourite in numerous soup recipes. Jacky says that when the bones are cooked for a long time, they release their collagen into the liquid, which becomes gelatinous, along with healthy amino acids, such as glycine and glutamine. All are said to be beneficial for the immune system, helpful for people with inflammatory bowel disease and lower bone density (especially menopausal women). Bone broth may also improve joint stiffness and pain caused by osteoarthritis.

Homemade vegetable stock is far healthier than store-bought. Peelings and other parts of vegetables that we might normally toss in the compost bin make for a nutrient-rich stock. Including vegetable stock in your diet helps you maintain a happy gut; it's a good source of vitamin A, important for healthy vision, along with being an antioxidant that can help towards eliminating free radicals and slowing down signs of aging. We often use veggie stock, like bone broth, as a base for soups and stews, though a cup of stock is also a delicious and highly nutritious drink.

When I am on my own for dinner I defrost a serving in a pot, throw in some vegetables and let them simmer until soft. My meal is ready by the time I have put on my pajamas, looking forward to a cozy night at home.

BONE BROTH

3 pounds (1½ kg) raw beef or chicken bones (grass-fed or organic)

2 tablespoons apple cider vinegar

2 carrots, chopped

2 stalks celery, chopped

1 onion, chopped

1 tablespoon sea salt (or to taste)

1 teaspoon whole peppercorns

3 bay leaves

2 cloves garlic, minced

1 bunch fresh parsley, chopped

Preheat the oven to 350°F (180°C). Place the bones in a roasting pan and roast for 30 minutes. Discard any excess fat.

Transfer the bones to a large stockpot. Pour plenty of water over the bones, fully submerging them, and add the vinegar. Let sit for 20 minutes. (The vinegar will help to release the nutrients in the bones.)

Add the carrots, celery, onion, salt, peppercorns and bay leaves to the pot. Cover and bring the broth to a gentle simmer over low heat. (Do not boil, as this will make the broth cloudy.) Simmer, still covered, for a minimum of 12 hours and up to 48 hours for beef bones or from 10 to 24 hours for chicken bones. (Remember to turn the stove off if you leave the house and at night, while you're asleep. The broth can sit with no heat under it overnight.) Foam may form on the surface of the soup; skim it off as it does.

During the last 30 minutes of cooking time, add the garlic and parsley.

Let the broth cool, then strain out and discard the solids. Store the broth in a large glass jar or portion-sized containers. The broth will keep in the fridge for up to 5 days or may be frozen for up to 6 months.

VEGETABLE STOCK

MAKES ABOUT 6 CUPS (1.5 L)

There really is no need to buy vegetable stock or broth at the store. Instead, all you need to do is collect your peelings and ends (from organic vegetables) and store them in the fridge, and whenever you have a few stray veggies lying about that are on their last legs, get out your stockpot!

2 carrots, chopped

2 stalks celery, chopped

1 onion, unpeeled, chopped

Peelings and ends from the above vegetables, plus whatever else you have saved up

1 tablespoon sea salt (or to taste)

1 teaspoon whole peppercorns

3 bay leaves

Fresh herbs, such as rosemary or thyme sprigs (optional)

2 cloves garlic, minced

1 bunch fresh parsley, chopped

In a large stockpot, combine all of the ingredients except the garlic and parsley. Pour water over the vegetables, fully submerging them. Bring to a gentle simmer over low heat; do not let boil. Simmer, covered, for at least 1 hour, or up to 3 hours if you're home for the day. During the last 30 minutes of cooking time, add the garlic and parsley.

Let the stock cool, then strain out and discard the solids. Store the stock in a large glass jar or portion-sized containers. The stock will keep in the fridge for up to 5 days, or may be frozen for up to 6 months.

TIP: The broth can also be simmered in a large covered casserole dish or pot in the oven on the lowest setting.

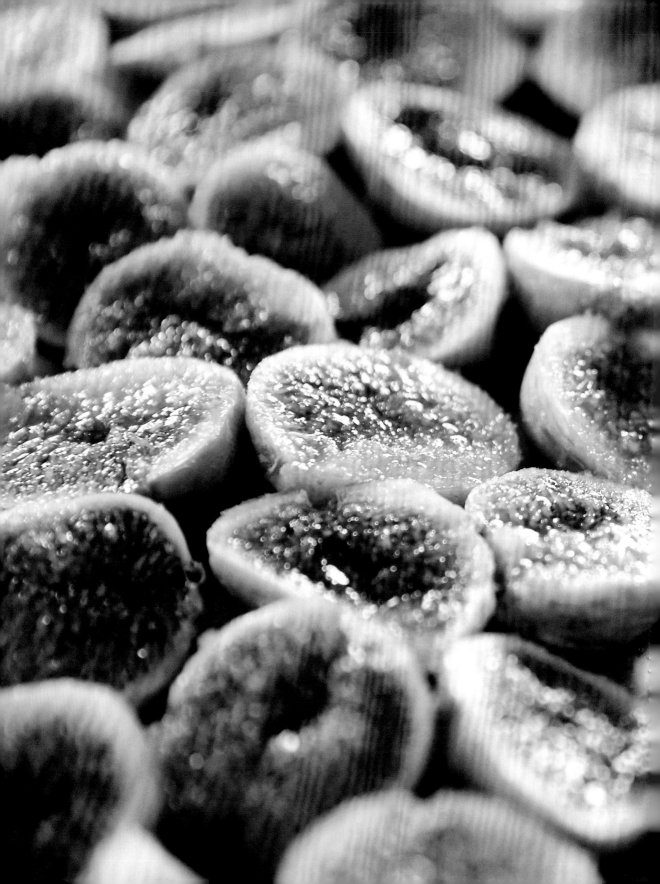

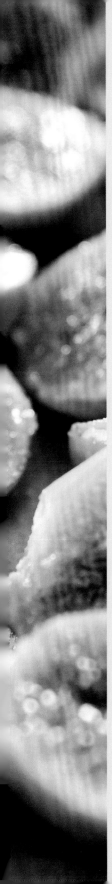

The Sweet Life

There's a longstanding Italian tradition of ending a meal with la frutta: a slice of watermelon, some Sicilian blood oranges or a perfectly ripe pear. The architect who was by my side during the renovation years, Bolko Von Schweinichen (such a delicious name), once explained this ritual over a working lunch. He had asked the waiter for "frutta, per favore," and to my astonishment, the waiter returned with half an apple on a plate and a small knife. Bolko continued to talk about the size of the new chimneys as I watched him delicately peel the apple, slice it into slim sections and enjoy it. Seeing my fascination, he told me that this was a valuable Italian lesson for dealing with the craving for a hit of sweetness at the end of a meal. The time it takes to peel and slice the apple reduces the craving, and the fruit satisfies the need for a sugary dessert, aids digestion and cleanses the palate.

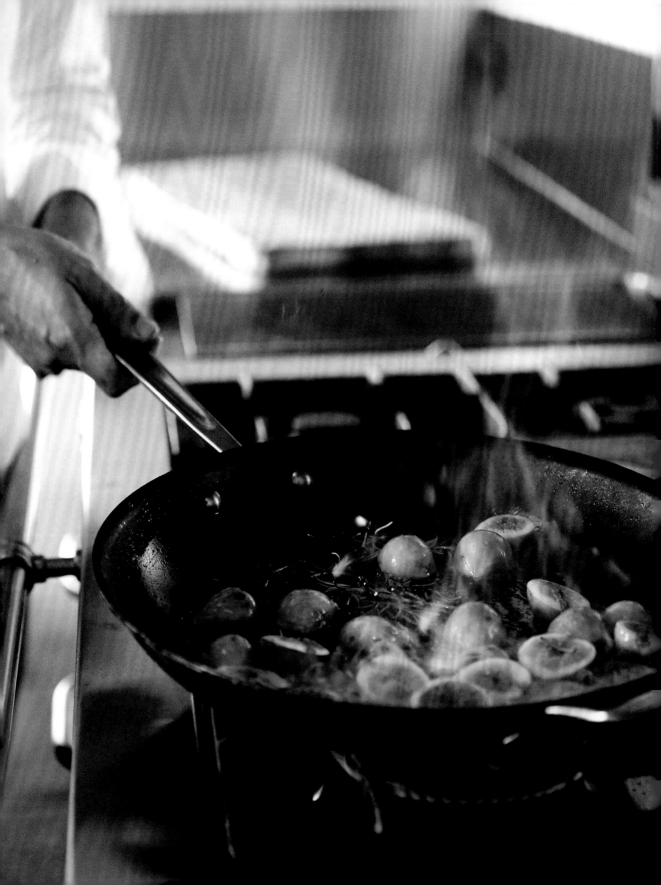

Italians do tuck into desserts when they are celebrating, often turning to recipes influenced by the cuisines of neighbouring countries. Favourites include a variety of *crostata*, or jam tarts, custard-based pies and the classic tiramisu. On a warm summer evening, ice cream lovers indulge in their beloved gelato, which seems to be as much about the social occasion as the marvels of Italian ice cream.

One of the delights of living in Tuscany is fig season. By September, the relentless summer sun begins to lose its harsh edge, and for three glorious weeks, plump figs ripen to the point of bursting open their skins—splitting like a fried sausage. Our figs have a natural green skin, soft and delicate, the flesh velvety red. We need to pick them before the insects invade or the fruit plops to the ground. Every day we roast or stew our harvest into a multitude of dishes. I am in seventh heaven when I devour them raw, the honey-like nectar oozing down my chin. But a large pan full, simmered in a cup of whisky or any alcohol (the only liquid added, no sugar necessary), becomes a bubbling, golden, sweet mess that I plop into sterilized jars and refrigerate for a future day so we can remember the joys of early autumn. We serve this thick jam with prosciutto and cheeses or dollop it on toast. The jam will only last about four months because no preservative or sugar is added, but it's rarely around that long at our place.

Another favourite dessert is roasted figs (a good source of fibre), which become sweeter as they cook. Slice the figs in half, place them on a baking sheet lined with parchment paper and roast at 350°F (180°C) for about ten minutes. Serve on a bed of bitter arugula with a crumbled tangy cheese—ricotta, blue cheese or feta—or a spoonful of natural yogurt.

Chef Francesco always includes a dessert after meals at the villa, a dash of sweetness to end the feast. Portions are tiny, a couple of mouthfuls. I recently shared a meal with friends in a large Italian-American restaurant in New Jersey, and the dessert that was served to me would easily have fed our entire Tuscan table of eighteen women. Much better to "have your dessert and eat it too," with the best possible ingredients and tiny portions.

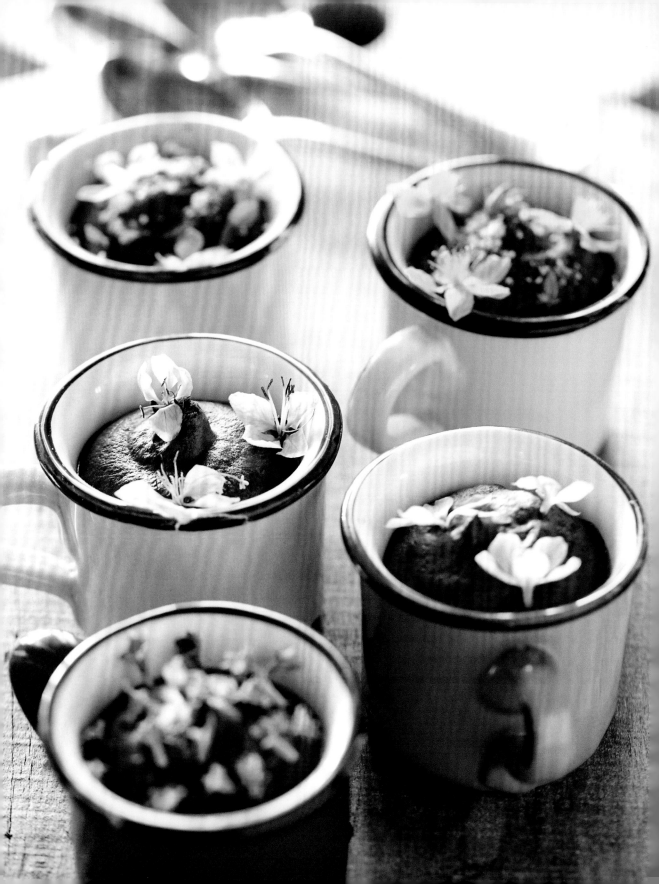

CHOCOLATE MOUSSE

SERVES 8

This is the go-to dessert at the villa—thick, rich and unforgettable.

4 cups whipping (heavy) cream
3 cups chopped dark chocolate (a little over 1 lb/500 g)
Icing (powdered) sugar
Edible flowers or fresh mint leaves

Pour the cream into a large bowl and whip with a whisk or electric mixer until stiff peaks form.

Place the chocolate in a microwave-safe bowl and microwave in 30-second intervals, stirring after each, until all the pieces are melted and the mixture is hot and smooth. (Alternatively, you can place the chocolate in a heatproof bowl and set it over a pot of gently boiling water, stirring regularly until melted and smooth.)

While the chocolate is still melted, quickly fold in the whipped cream using a spatula, mixing gently and gradually until the mousse is fluffy and soft. Using a piping bag (or a zip-lock bag with a small hole cut in the corner), pipe the mousse into individual serving dishes and refrigerate for at least 3 hours, until the mousse is chilled and the texture firm.

When ready to serve, dust each portion with a little icing sugar and decorate with flowers or mint (or however your creative juices inspire you).

JACKY SAYS

Chocolate is a double-edged sword: too much and it can be an unhealthy choice that goes straight to the hips, but a little now and again can be a wholesome treat. The healthiest chocolate to consume contains 70 to 80 percent cacao, which is pure chocolate from crushed beans. Cacao provides small amounts of fibre and protein as well as fat, and is rich in polyphenols, which have antioxidant and anti-inflammatory effects.

Nutritionally, pure chocolate is quite extraordinary, as it contains small amounts of essential minerals such as magnesium, copper, iron, potassium, zinc and calcium, and even a little vitamin K. One small bite of the good stuff, savoured mindfully, can stop the craving for the overly sweetened processed chocolate we are all so familiar with.

Love Your Gut

In the last few years, the gut has become a central concern of all diets, whether you're eating to maintain your health, to lose weight or to de-stress your system. And for good reason. On the whole, the Mediterranean diet is anti-inflammatory. Nutritionally balanced, home-cooked meals, full of fibre and diverse ingredients, reduce inflammation, keeping the gut in good working order. The Italians have got it right: our guts thrive on a diverse and balanced diet.

The gut also appreciates it when we give ourselves time to eat and time to digest. Avoid grab-and-go meals by planning and preparing foods in advance so you always have a healthy option at the ready. A few hours in the kitchen on a Sunday afternoon can set you up for the week ahead. Make a batch of soup, ready to warm up after a long workday. Stock the fridge with containers of cooked rice, chickpeas or spelt, some roast chicken, avocadoes, steamed beets and broccoli, and a couple of baked sweet potatoes. Having it all ready to go means you can create "fast food" in your own house. And being prepared also makes it easier to avoid both snacking and the impulsive high-fat, sugary and salty food choices that spike our blood sugar and lead to an irritated gut and low energy.

Mangia Bene. Eat Well

Despite my many years in Italy, I am still intrigued by the eating habits of this country. I do believe that the way they eat, and the way they eat together, has a lot to do with Italian longevity. Their meals are not fussy, relying on ingredients that are fresh and in season. They rarely snack, and they don't gulp their food on the run. Italians always take the time to savour and discuss what they're eating.

How to Bring Tuscany Home

- Eat fresh, in-season, locally grown food as much as possible.
- Take a lesson from your granny: buy in bulk when fruits and vegetables are in season and preserve, freeze or ferment the excess. Try your best to waste very little.
- Avoid eating packaged foods whenever possible; the less you eat of these highly processed foods, the better.
- Buy organic vegetables when you can.
- Support local farmers. Many will deliver fresh seasonal veggies to your doorstep.
- Eat the alphabet of fruits and vegetables, covering the spectrum of magnificent natural colours.
- Be prepared: spend a few hours a week organizing meals for the days ahead.
- Take the time to enjoy each meal, and reduce snacking as much as possible.
- Hail the leaves! Move on from commercial bags of lettuce and try different fresh varieties of leafy green vegetables.
- Lose your fear of carbs, but choose healthy whole grains.
- Watch out for hidden sugar: always read labels.
- Aim for a plant-based diet with small amounts of meat and fish (if you are not vegetarian or vegan).
- Eat fermented food daily.
- Enjoy dairy, but in limited amounts, and choose the very best quality.
- Ensure olive oil is extra virgin and is actually produced in the country credited on the label.

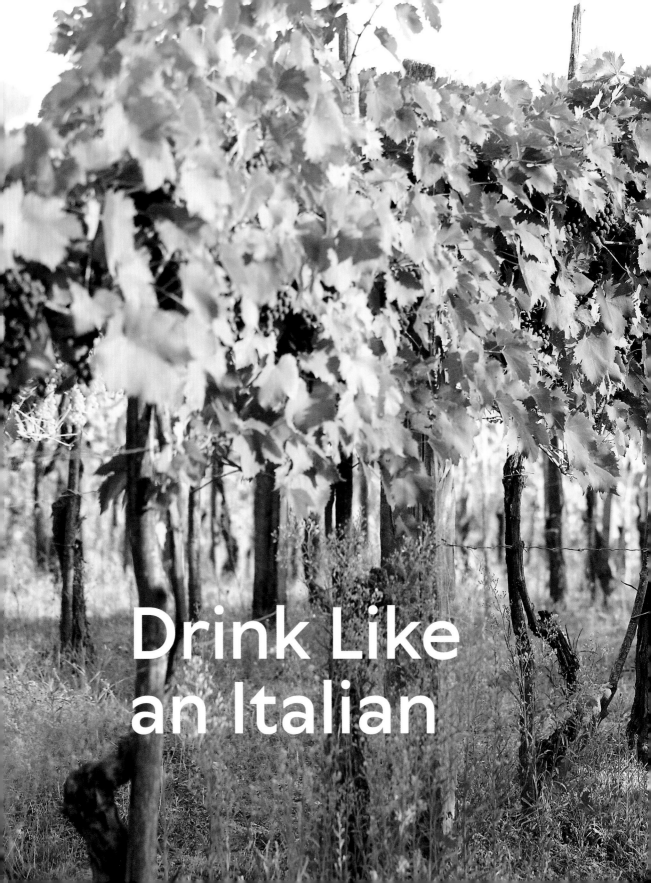

Drink Like
an Italian

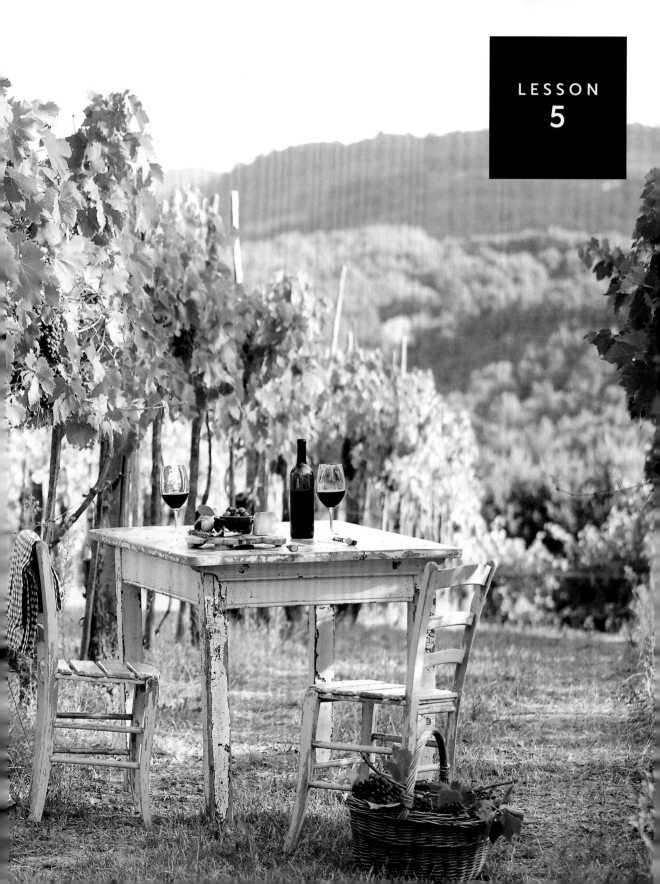

Sip in Style

IT TOOK JUST ONE TRIP TO ITALY for me to realize that the Italian drinking culture is a far cry from my own. First, a café and a bar in Italy are one and the same. Life here is a social event from sunrise to late at night. People go to coffee shops in the mornings, just as they do where I come from, but here you will never see people clutching extra-large takeout cups full of mochas, caramel-flavoured macchiatos, chestnut praline lattes or gigantic Americanos as they head to work. Instead, you'll notice patrons, all of whom seem to be on the best of terms with the proprietor, taking their shots of espresso in little china cups as they stand at the bar, or people settling in to enjoy a small latte and a pastry at a table while they chat with a friend. You might also spy a farmer knocking back a grappa alongside a shot of coffee before he heads off for the fields on his tractor. At the end of an evening, it is rare to witness drunken revellers spewing out of the bars, as they do at closing time in England and North America. It is an Italian pastime to enjoy an *aperitivo* at the end of the day—a single glass with nibbles—followed by a small amount of wine with dinner. I have to admit that when Hans and I first started being invited to the local communal meals, a collection of empty wine bottles would accumulate at my end of the table while my neighbours would still be nursing their first glass. It has taken me awhile to learn to drink like an Italian, but it is a much healthier alternative!

Italy is the largest producer of wine after France, yet Italians are not known for heavy drinking. They enjoy alcohol in moderation as an everyday custom, and tend to view wine as an accompaniment to food. When guests come to my house, they are immediately handed a glass of something wonderful. I am still not used to the fact that when you go to an Italian friend's for a party, you can stand around for an hour longingly ogling the wine bottle, as you patiently wait for dinner to be served. Your hosts chat away charmingly, never thinking to ask if you would like a drink. It is a tradition I am trying to embrace, but I do like to be offered a drink as I'm hanging up my coat!

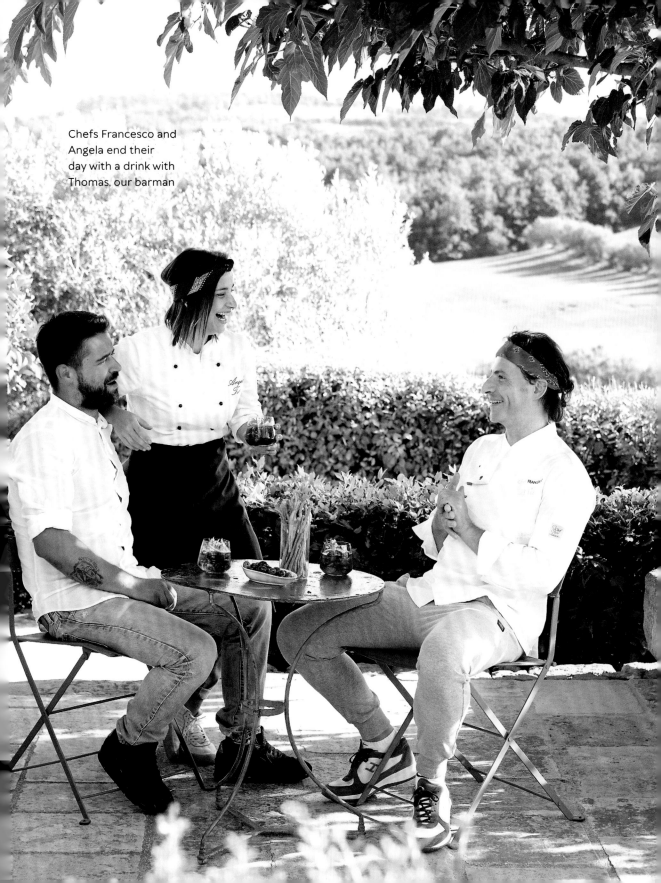

Chefs Francesco and
Angela end their
day with a drink with
Thomas, our barman

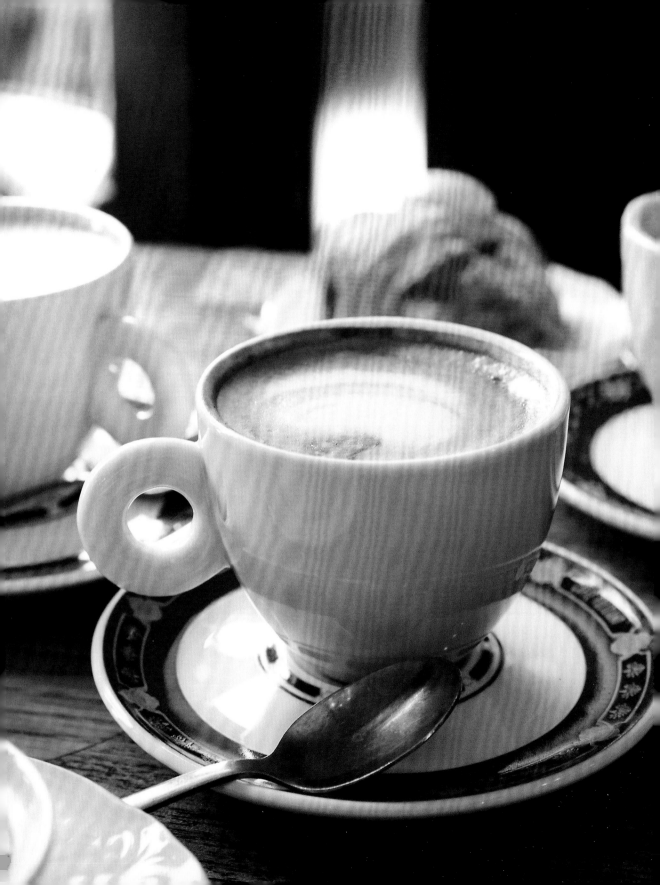

Coffee Culture

Regardless of the constant health studies on the pros and cons of drinking coffee, there is no prising Italians away from this morning ritual. As a nation they drink about three cups a day, just like the rest of us, but as I mentioned, there's a big difference in the size of the cups, the quality of the beans and how coffee is made!

And then there is the way they drink it, which is never grab-and-go. Outside of the main tourist cities, you will never see a mass coffee chain. Local bars serve good-quality coffee in porcelain or glass cups, never paper or Styrofoam. There are many ways to drink your coffee on offer, now emulated in cafés around the world. Espressos are accompanied by a tiny glass of water to cleanse the palate, so you can taste the richness of the bean. (Jacky points out that coffee is a diuretic, so drinking it with a glass of water helps you stay hydrated, especially in the summer months.) Italians drink cappuccinos or lattes only as a breakfast drink. Tourists who order one in the afternoon or at the end of an evening meal might be shocked by the passionate response from the waiter, who may even point out to them this is *not* the right thing to do! Since milky drinks take longer to digest, it actually does make sense to enjoy a latte or cappuccino in the morning, which also gives your body time to work off the calories. Not to mention that sugar from the milk's lactose gives us a wake-up boost of energy on top of the kick from the caffeine.

But setting aside how and when we drink it, is coffee good or bad for us? It turns out that drinking good-quality coffee in moderation has numerous health benefits; some researchers have correlated increased longevity with moderate use. But we all react differently to caffeine, with some of us being more sensitive than others. We need to truly understand how our own bodies respond to this stimulant. When our guests share with us that they're suffering from anxiety, insomnia, restlessness or irritability and we ask how many cups of coffee they drink each day, they often respond, "Oh, coffee doesn't bother me! I can drink as much as I want, when I want." Really? If you don't sleep so well at night, wake up groggy and need gallons of the stuff to get into the swing of the day, you may be drinking just a bit too much coffee!

JACKY SAYS

Coffee stimulates the nervous system, giving you a short-term boost in brain function. Some studies have found that coffee has positive effects on the liver, provides some protection against type 2 diabetes, Alzheimer's and Parkinson's, and may be associated with maintaining a lower body weight. There are more beneficial antioxidants in lighter roasted beans than in dark ones. The way espresso is made, by shooting boiling steam through freshly ground coffee, is thought to release more of the rich coffee oils into the shot than are reaped by brewing American-style coffee.

However, too much caffeine, or coffee drunk too late in the day, can interfere with sleep and cause upset stomach, tremors and palpitations. In addition, people who suffer from anxiety or stress should avoid coffee, because the excess caffeine exacerbates these conditions by raising cortisol (stress hormone) levels.

Be sure to check out the quality of your daily coffee. If you buy your coffee at the same spot every day, ask what kind of bean they use. Italy does not grow coffee beans; the great quality comes from how Italian coffee companies roast and blend the imported beans. At the villa, we're lucky enough to have one of those fancy coffee machines you see in upscale coffee shops, and our guests love the taste of the organic Italian coffee we serve. Each morning, we encourage it to hiss and splurt its nectar into countless cups. I have to say, we make an astounding cappuccino. Good-quality coffee can be found everywhere, and once you have educated your taste buds, it is hard to go back to the commercial stuff.

So drink your coffee the Italian way: find a café that is proud of the quality of their coffee and enjoy the ritual, using your morning cup as an excuse to pause, to savour the experience and maybe also to visit with a friend. It is a marvellous way to start the day.

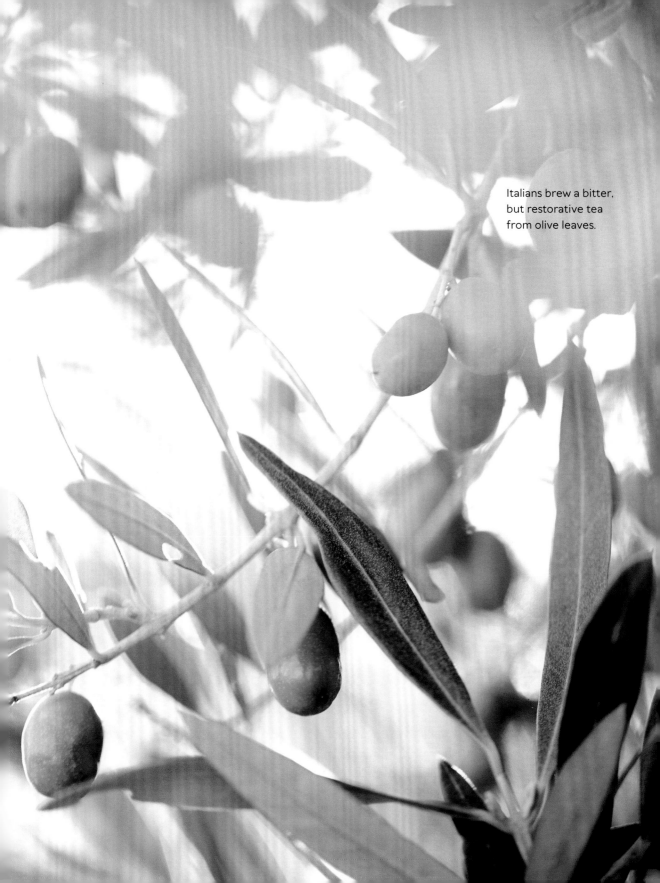

Italians brew a bitter, but restorative tea from olive leaves.

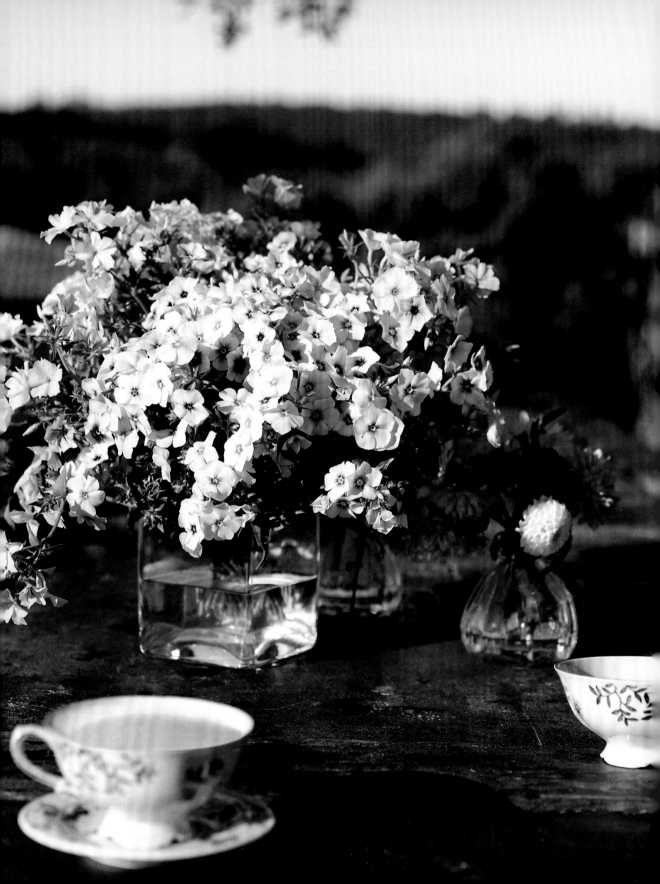

Tea, the Italian Way

As a Brit, I always have a pot of tea brewing in my home. Where I grew up, a cuppa was the answer to every life crisis and was offered to everyone who dropped in. In Italy, although tea-drinking is slowly growing in popularity, Italians regard tea as more of a healing tonic, made by steeping a variety of herbs and leaves in hot water. At the villa, our teas are in our medicine cabinet. We make all kinds of teas from the fresh herbs, shrubs and trees that grow around us, and we harvest big bunches in season to dry and use all winter long.

If you want to try any of the suggestions below, the rule of thumb is to use about a teaspoon of dried herbs per cup, or two or three times that if the herbs are fresh. With fresh herbs especially, I don't mind if they float around in my cup, but you can also put the dried or fresh leaves in an individual strainer or use a teapot. Boil freshly drawn cold water—if it's filtered, even better—because the oxygen helps to release the herbal flavours. (Your tea won't taste anywhere near as good if you reboil the water that's been sitting in the kettle.) Never pour boiling water directly onto the tea leaves: it will scorch them and damage the natural flavours. Either let the kettle sit for a couple of minutes after it has boiled, then pour the water, or douse the bag or leaves with a tiny amount of cold water before you pour in the hot water. The longer the steep (five minutes is a good rule of thumb), the more nutrients and oils are drawn out into the water; be careful, though, because too long a steep can turn the tea bitter.

A note about tea bags. They are convenient and have their place, but I have to say that nothing beats tea made in a teapot with loose leaves that have released their flavour and natural goodness. If you prefer tea bags, try to use plastic-free, unbleached ones.

SOME VILLA TEA FAVOURITES

FENNEL: Fennel tea supports digestion and eases bloating. The delicate flavour is immediately relaxing. We use a tablespoon of fennel seeds per cup (more than the usual amount for a dried herbal tea) and also add fennel fronds—the frilly green bits on top of the bulb—from the garden when they are in season. We let this one steep for ten minutes instead of the usual five.

CHAMOMILE: The oils found in the delicate chamomile flower release disease-fighting, anti-inflammatory antioxidants that support sleep and tranquility and aid digestion.

SAGE: The sage we harvest around the villa gets as big as a shrub; with a lovely silver-grey leaf, it's one of more than nine hundred types of sage that grow around the world. The Romans used sage tea to aid digestion, and it's a popular remedy in Tuscany to help soothe coughs and colds and to treat certain skin diseases. We offer it to guests who are experiencing symptoms of menopause; a cup of sage tea relieves night sweats because it helps balance the hormones.

MINT, one of the most flavourful and familiar of herbs, grows like a weed around the property. We recommend a cup of fresh mint tea after dinner, to cleanse the palate and settle the stomach.

GREEN TEA is thought to have the biggest health benefits of all the teas. It is an antioxidant, protects the brain from free radical damage and is appreciated for its levels of L-theanine, a non-essential amino acid. My favourite green tea comes as "pearls" infused with jasmine. Putting a spoonful of these tiny rolled-up leaves into a glass teapot and watching them unfurl in the hot water is my own personal tea ceremony each morning.

GINGER is used mostly in Christmas baking in Italian kitchens, but it is also grated into hot water as a drink that settles the stomach and supports the detoxification of the liver and the immune system. Ginger is an age-old remedy for healthy circulation.

LAVENDER: Not only does lavender release a relaxing, beautiful perfume, but a tea made from its flowers is anti-inflammatory and full of antioxidants. Steep a couple of teaspoons of lavender flowers in a two-cup teapot for five minutes and inhale, then sip: this brew will help relieve stress and anxiety. A perfect bedtime drink.

ROSEHIP: There are banks of wild roses along the back roads here. Once the petals have fallen off, around September, the deep red rosehips that form are used to treat a range of conditions. Rosehip tea has a high concentration of vitamin C and is said to significantly reduce pain levels for those suffering with arthritis.

THYME: Wild thyme grows all around us here, but it also grows well in pots and is easily found year-round in the supermarket. This deliciously scented herb adds rich flavour to soups, vinaigrettes and stews, and thyme tea with a spoonful of honey added helps soothe irritating coughs and bronchitis.

OLIVE LEAF: Tea made from olive leaves is bitter, but it can be sweetened with honey to make it more palatable. It is an acquired taste, but a cup a day is fantastic during a detox, as the oils from the leaves have properties that help lower blood pressure and improve cholesterol levels, and are a healthy supplement for those with type 2 diabetes. After a night out when I've eaten a lot and had more than one glass of wine, I often drink a cup of olive leaf tea before I fall asleep.

ROSEMARY: The aroma of rosemary tea alone is a mood enhancer, and a cup made from the waxy, needle-like leaves has many benefits, especially anti-inflammatory effects. Rosemary oils can improve memory, help alleviate joint and muscle pain, boost the immune system and even help with hair loss.

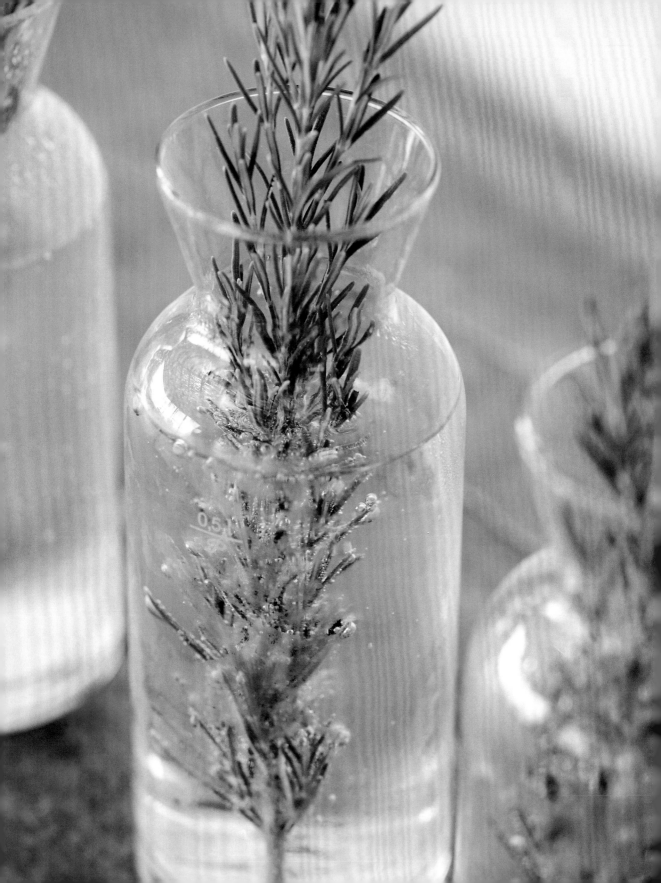

Replenish with Water

There are numerous natural springs around here, which you can always locate by the sight of a person bent over, surrounded by large containers. The Tuscans know where the good stuff is: pure mountain water tastes better than anything from the tap or a bottle.

With Tuscan summer temperatures hitting record highs in recent years, we never forget to drink lots of water. But good health depends on proper hydration, wherever you live. If you suffer from regular headaches, low energy, stomach problems, difficulty concentrating, sugar cravings, skin breakouts or bowel issues, try increasing your water consumption before you head for the medicine cabinet. It just might make the difference.

It can be challenging to drink enough water every day; there are even apps available to remind us. The way it works best for me is to pour my daily quota (I use eight glasses as my benchmark, on Jacky's advice) into a couple of jugs in the morning and leave them in plain sight. When I can see them, I remember to drink them dry!

Some people don't like the taste of plain water. If you're one of them, try adding the juice of a squeezed lemon, lime or orange (or all three) to your water jug. A tablespoon of grated ginger is also refreshing and tasty. If you prefer to drink sparkling water, try diluting it by half with plain water. Too much fizz is apparently not good for the bones.

Monitor your pee to check if you're getting enough water. Jacky says it should be a pale Prosecco colour by midday, not golden yellow (although golden yellow is normal first thing in the morning).

One idea many of our guests take home from the villa is to pop a large sprig of rosemary into a jug or water bottle. It looks beautiful, for one thing, but water infused with rosemary is also good for us, as the ancients knew. (See rosemary tea, above, for details on the health benefits of rosemary.) We have hedges of rosemary around the villa, and it grows successfully in most places, though it does die in the winter in northern climates. Still, all summer long, whether in a pot or in the garden, you can harvest rosemary, rinse the branches well and infuse your daily water with the oils that seep from the leaves. Unadulterated goodness.

So What About That Glass or Two of Wine?

Each year, even with all I've learned from living in Tuscany, I am among the revellers who have too much fun over the holidays. What can I say? I love people and I love parties. As a result, every January I follow along with all the other detoxers and abstain for the whole month. Boring, yes, but after a few days, boy do I feel good! I sleep through the night, eight solid hours. I lose the puffy face, inches disappear from my waist and my joints feel less stiff. I am perfectly happy not drinking any alcohol—until the next get-together with friends, romantic dinner with my hubby or the *piazza* beckoning me on a sunny day. Although I do reap the benefits from abstaining, I know I can never give up the joy of drinking a glass or two of wine, so except for those darn holidays, I try to follow in the steady steps of my Tuscan neighbours.

I actually find nothing quite so confusing as trying to weigh the pros and cons of drinking alcohol. In part, I find it tricky because people react differently to it. For some, alcohol is an addiction that wrecks them physically and emotionally. Others have no trouble at all sticking to a noble glass of wine with a fine meal, appreciating it as a simple pleasure. Jacky tells me that 20 percent of the alcohol we drink is absorbed through the wall of the stomach into the bloodstream—in other words, pretty much right after you swallow it—where it can stimulate the production of a neurotransmitter, gamma-aminobutyric acid (GABA), that relaxes us. That's why alcohol helps us be more social. But the alcohol we drink is processed by the liver, and when we drink in excess, we stress this vital organ, creating numerous health problems. Drinking also wreaks havoc with our sugar levels, affecting our energy levels, our weight and our sleep.

Yet Italy, a country of wine drinkers (even in moderation, as a nation they drink a lot of wine) has one of the longest-living populations on the planet. Some scientists say that red wine, in particular, has a beneficial effect in moderation because it contains resveratrol, a natural chemical found in the skin and pips of the red grape.

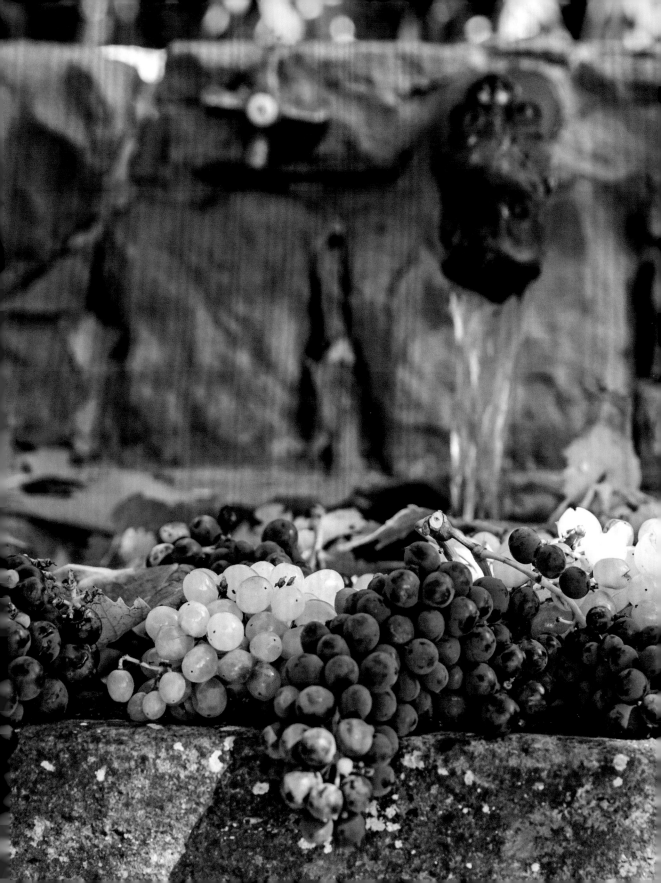

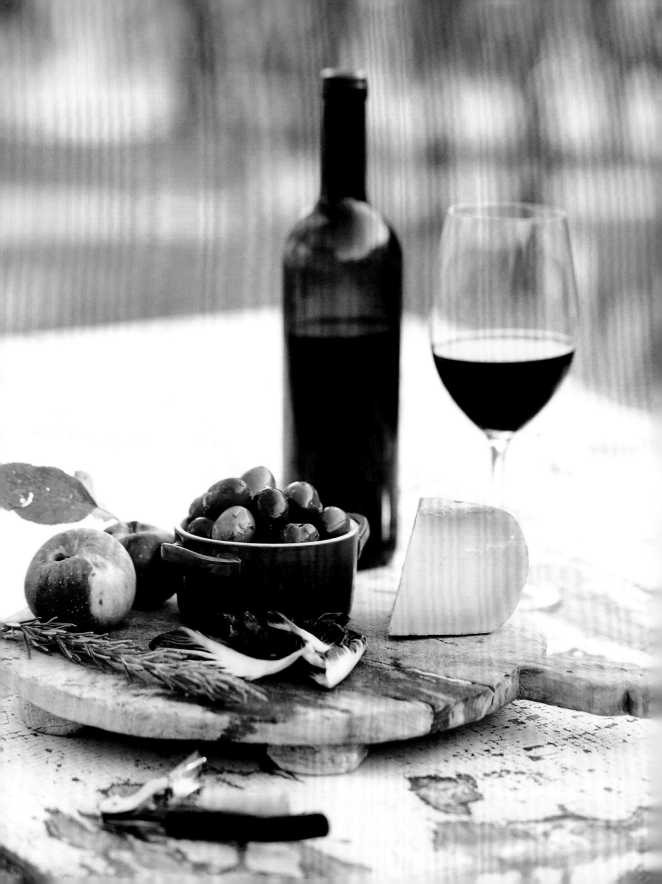

Jacky has dug into this claim and says some studies have shown that the quantities of resveratrol in red wine are too low to have any impact on our health. Until we have absolute proof, though, I think I'm going to put my money on the scientists who say it's good for us—but believing, along with the Italians, that the secret to the beneficial impact of wine lies in enjoying at most a glass or two each day. The real value may simply lie in the social enjoyment: being relaxed and happy while sipping a marvellous glass of *vino* in the company of people you connect with.

So instead of glugging it back, let's all drink like the Italians do. I am trying so hard!

The Marvellous *Aperitivo*

The *aperitivo* is, above all, a warm affair. It can be, and is, many things: a leisurely pre-dinner drink, awakening the taste buds for the meal to come; a chance to relax when the workday is finished; a catch-up with friends. After a long day filming my design shows, I loved to lounge on my front lawn on a summer evening, still in my paint-splattered overalls, chatting with my close buddies Christina and Helen over a bottle of wine or a gin and tonic as we watched the kids playing soccer on the patch of grass outside the nearby town hall. The break in the daily routine, along with the pleasure we took in each other's company, gave us the energy boost we needed before we tackled what we called the "witching hour": wrestling the kids into the bath and then into bed. Priceless times. Nothing has really changed, as now, when all our chores are done, Hans and I hike up to the ancient village for an *aperitivo*, a glass of Prosecco with the locals and newfound friends—or, if we are feeling a little more daring, a Negroni—along with the lovely free snacks the bar serves.

Following are a couple of recipes that might inspire you to take a break with some loved ones and friends in the spirit of the *aperitivo*. A note for non-drinkers: the company is the point here; you can toast the table just as well with a glass of sparkling water. (I add a little grated ginger and a squeeze of lime to mine.)

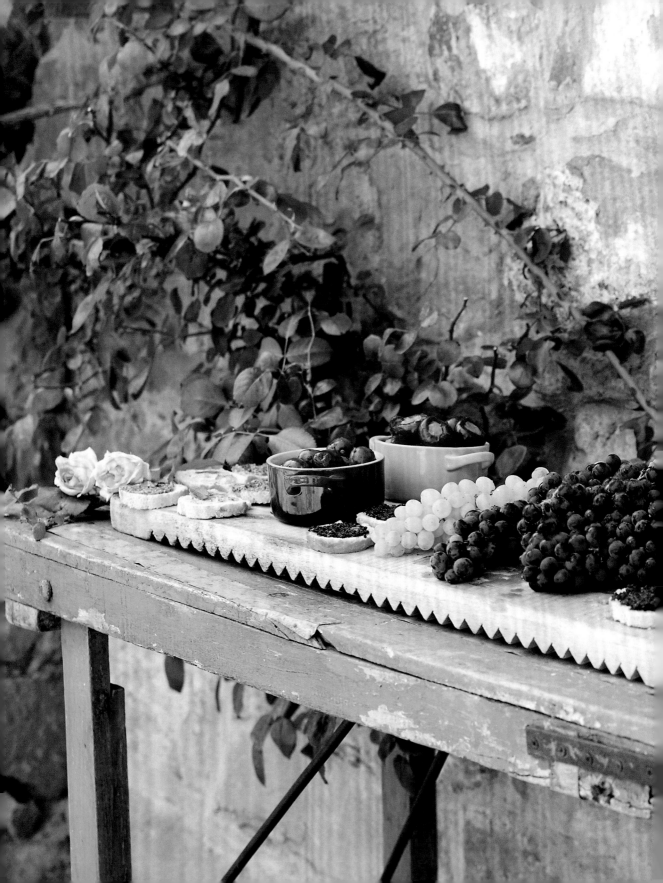

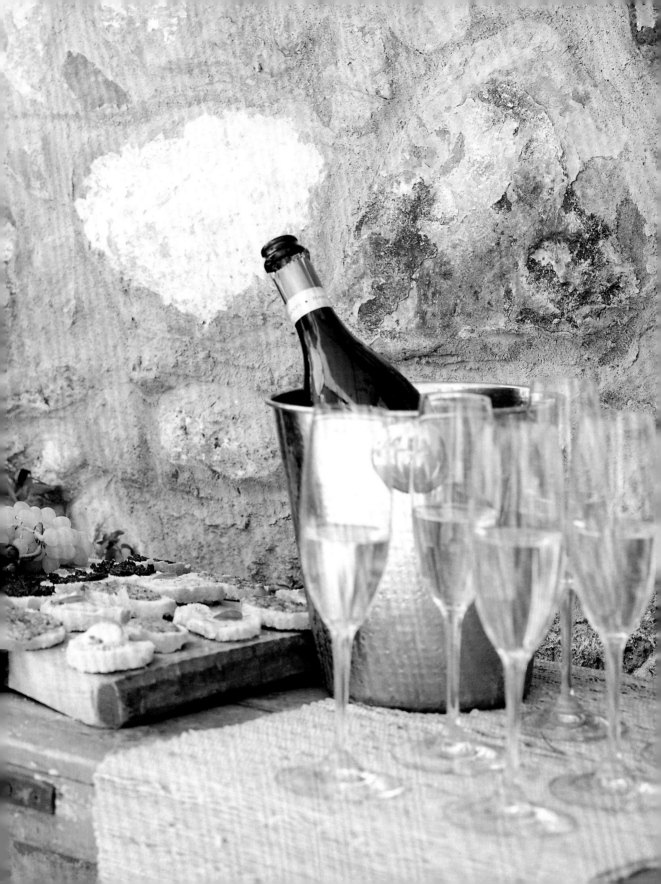

CROSTINI, THREE WAYS

SERVES 6 TO 8

PESTO TOPPING:

½ cup pine nuts

2 cloves garlic, peeled and smashed with the flat side of a knife

4 cups fresh basil leaves

½ cup extra virgin olive oil

Salt and freshly ground black pepper to taste

½ cup freshly grated Parmesan cheese

MUSHROOM TOPPING:

2 tablespoons extra virgin olive oil

8 ounces (250 g) cremini or button mushrooms, finely chopped

1 tablespoon unsalted butter

2 cloves garlic, minced

Leaves from 1 sprig fresh rosemary, minced

Pinch of freshly ground pepper

Pinch of salt

TOASTS:

Favourite bread for small toasts or Italian crostini (could be a crunchy baguette or focaccia), cut into ½-inch slices

Extra virgin olive oil (you'll need about ½ cup total)

Freshly ground pepper

Coarse salt

GORGONZOLA TOPPING:

7 ounces (200 g) creamy gorgonzola cheese

Honey

Fresh sage leaves

Preheat the oven to 425°F (220°C).

To make the pesto: In a small frying pan, over medium heat, lightly toast the pine nuts for 2 minutes, stirring constantly.

Add the garlic, basil, olive oil, salt and pepper to a food processor fitted with a steel blade. Toss in the toasted pine nuts and process until combined. Spoon the mixture into a bowl and gently stir in the Parmesan cheese. Set aside.

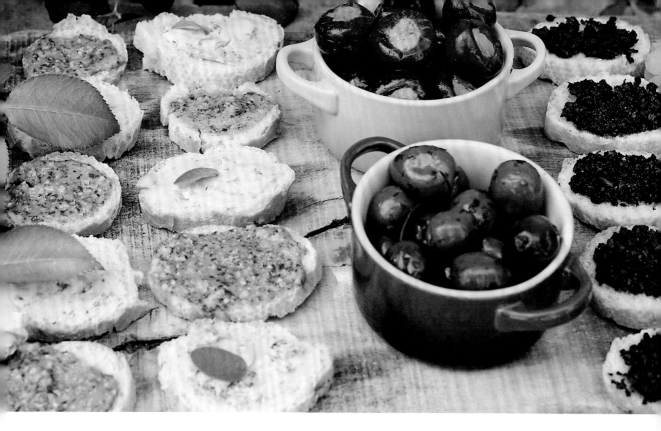

For the mushrooms: In a large frying pan, heat the olive oil over medium-high heat. Add the mushrooms and cook for about 8 minutes, until they are softened and releasing their juices. Lower the heat to medium-low and add the butter, garlic, rosemary, pepper and salt. Cook for another 20 minutes, low and slow, until the mushrooms are browned and a little crispy. Don't stir too often—maybe once halfway through.

For the toasts: When your pesto and mushrooms are ready, brush the bread slices with olive oil and sprinkle with pepper and coarse salt. Toast in the preheated oven for about 6 minutes, until warmed through but not crisp. Check often to make sure they don't burn.

To serve: Dollop a third of the toasts with a teaspoon of pesto each. Top another third with spoonfuls of the mushroom mixture. Spread the last third with roughly a tablespoon of gorgonzola each, drizzle with honey and decorate each with a single sage leaf. Yum.

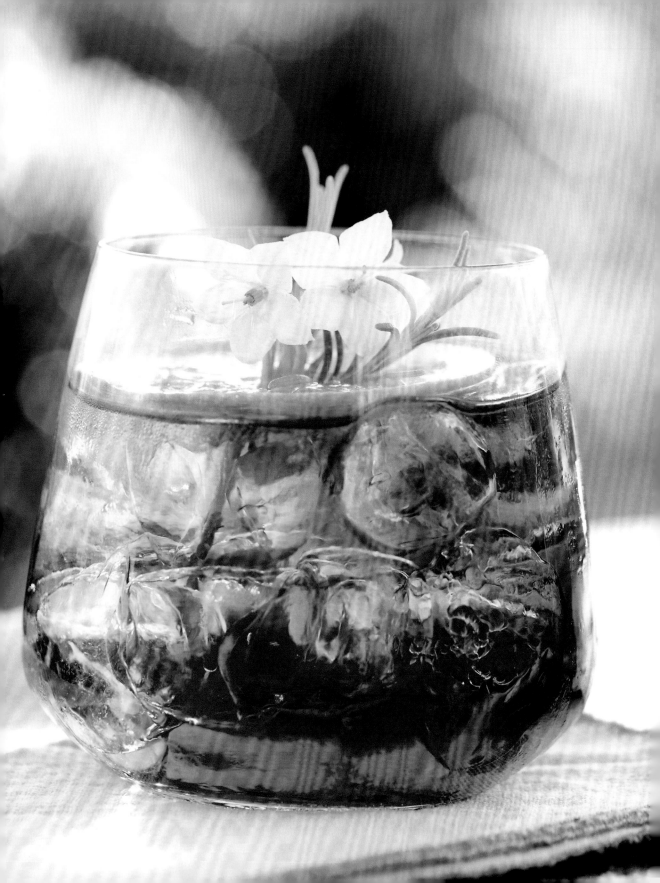

APEROL SPRITZ, VILLA RENIELLA-STYLE

Now for a very special *aperitivo*-time cocktail. Luminous in colour, this classic Italian drink is, for me, the taste of warm summer evenings. You can make a simple version, in which you dilute aromatic, citrusy Aperol with Prosecco and a splash of sparkling water (2 parts Aperol, 3 parts Prosecco and 1 part sparkling water), pour over ice and garnish with orange slices. Or you can try our version, created by Thomas, our beloved barman.

FOR ONE:

2 ounces (60 ml) Aperol
¼ ounce (7 ml) lychee liqueur
1 ounce (30 ml) cranberry juice
½ ounce (15 ml) orange juice
2 to 3 ounces (60 to 90 ml) Prosecco, or to taste
1 orange slice

In a large, round wineglass, stir together the first four ingredients, then top up with the Prosecco. Garnish with an orange slice or edible flowers. (You can also serve this drink over ice.)

FOR A CROWD:

16 ounces (500 ml) Aperol
2 ounces (60 ml) lychee liqueur
8 ounces (250 ml) cranberry juice
4 ounces (125 ml) orange juice
16 ounces (500 ml) Prosecco
8 orange slices

Use the same technique as with a single cocktail, but use a pitcher.

Limoncello Laughs

It may seem bizarre, at a retreat aimed at recharging burned-out bodies and minds and living with optimal health, to feature a workshop on the art of making limoncello, the beloved Italian *digestivo*. But getting together to learn how to make this bright and sunny drink always leaves our guests beaming—and I receive lots of wonderful photos from women who hold their own limoncello-making parties after they get home. Mission accomplished! The drink is delicious, but the joy is found in making it *together*.

Traditionally from southern Italy—where the locals like to proclaim that their family recipe, always a closely guarded secret, makes a more delicious drink than their neighbours'—limoncello can be made anywhere you have a bunch of lemons and the desire. Just gather a large bowl, a few glass bottles of different shapes and sizes with tight lids, several graters and peelers, and the ingredients listed below, which are enough to make about 8 cups (2 L) of limoncello. You could even buy a pack of sticky labels and customize a design to commemorate the "vintage." Next, invite a few friends and tell each one to bring another person, so you'll end up with double the friends packed into your kitchen. Before the party starts, make sure you sterilize the bottles and lids (by washing them in the dishwasher or boiling them in water for 5 minutes) so they're ready to go. When the guests arrive, crank up the music and divide them into peelers, graters and squeezers.

However you organize, the group will create a little heaven on earth with the recipe below—it's silky, sweet and tangy, like lemon cake in a bottle, only with a kick. What with all the peeling, grating, squeezing, stirring and taste-testing, I guarantee a riotous time. And everyone gets to go home with their own bottle or two!

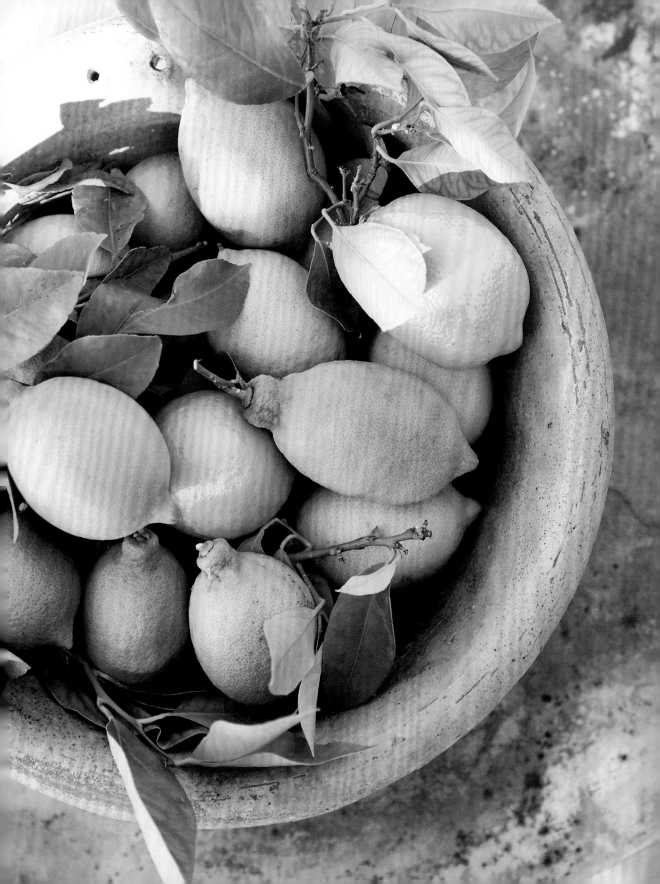

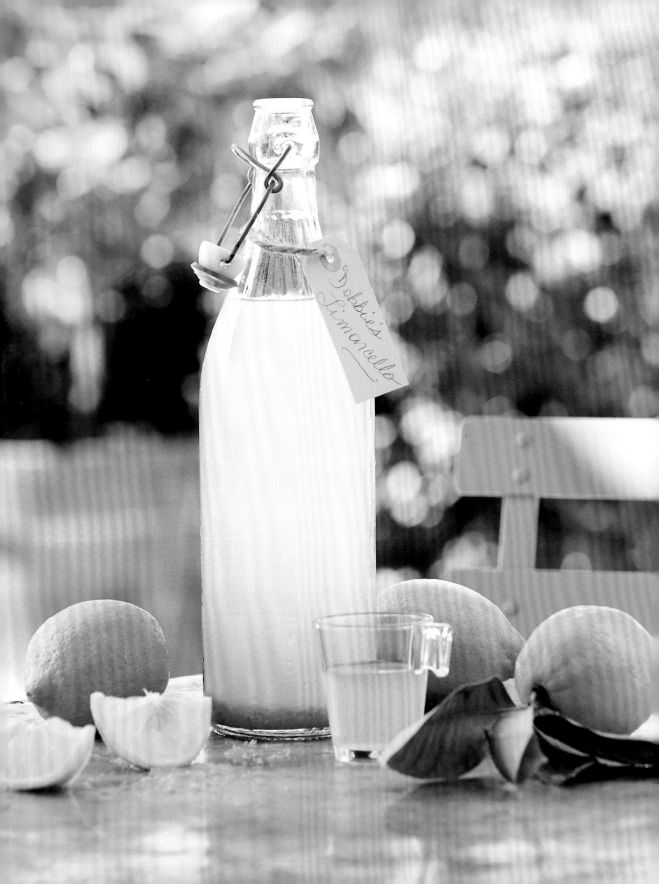

LIMONCELLO

FOR ONE BATCH:

15 to 20 lemons (unwaxed)

2¼ cups granulated sugar

26-ounce (750 ml) bottle of grain alcohol

7 ounces (200 ml) unflavoured vodka

Peel some of the lemons, taking care to avoid the white pith, until you have 1 cup or so of thin strips. In a medium saucepan, combine the sugar and 3 cups of water. Add the lemon peel. Heat on medium, stirring occasionally, until the sugar dissolves. Turn off the heat and let the simple syrup you've made sit for awhile to allow the oils from the lemon peel to flavour it.

Zest some of the remaining lemons with a fine grater until you have about 3 cups of zest. (Remember, the lemons must be unwaxed—you don't want wax in the drink.) Then cut all of the peeled and zested lemons in half and squeeze out all the juice, removing any pips.

In a large bowl, combine 2 cups of the zest with the grain alcohol, vodka and lemon juice. Strain the simple syrup and discard the peel, then add the syrup to the bowl. Stir well and taste! If the limoncello tastes too strong, add more water until it suits you. If it tastes too sweet, squeeze more lemons and add the juice.

Add a tablespoon or so of the remaining lemon zest to each of your sterilized glass bottles and carefully pour in the limoncello. Cap the bottles, wipe them down if they've become sticky, add a label to each and present them to your guests. Let the limoncello steep in the refrigerator for at least a month to develop its flavour. Then crack the bottle open and enjoy! (Afterwards, keep it in the freezer.)

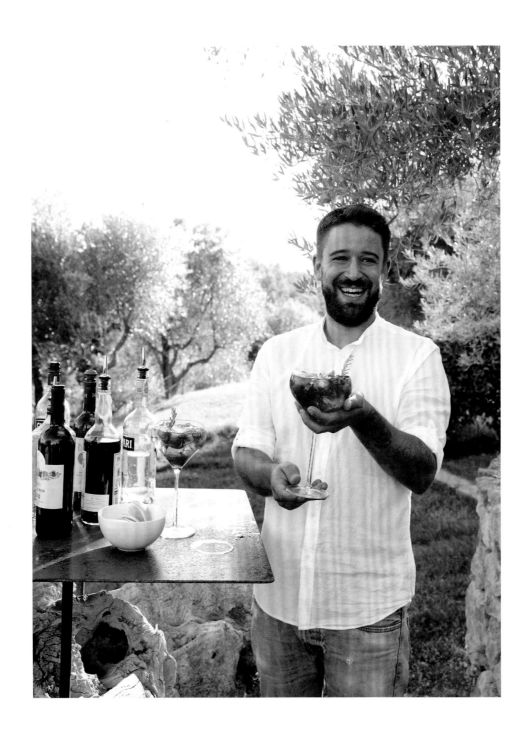

JOY

How to Bring Tuscany Home

- Make a habit of sitting down in the morning, even for a few minutes, to enjoy a coffee and get your thoughts together for the day, rather than drinking your coffee on the go.
- Cleanse your palate with a glass of water before and after drinking coffee. This is also a good way to rehydrate.
- Find a regular coffee place that has the best-quality beans.
- Drink milky coffee before lunch.
- Try loose-leaf tea rather than using tea bags. Avoid white tea bags, as most have been bleached.
- Experiment with different fresh herbal teas, especially to help with sleep and indigestion. Fresh herbs steeped in a pot can be so much more enjoyable than herbal tea bags.
- Make it a habit to drink plenty of water. Up your intake to at least eight large glasses a day. Pour the quantity you intend to drink into a jug and keep it in sight, so you don't forget.
- Flavour your water with lemon, lime, orange, ginger or even rosemary.
- Drink alcohol like an Italian—in moderation!
- Sip and linger, watching the people and life around you, rather than gulping down your favourite cocktail.

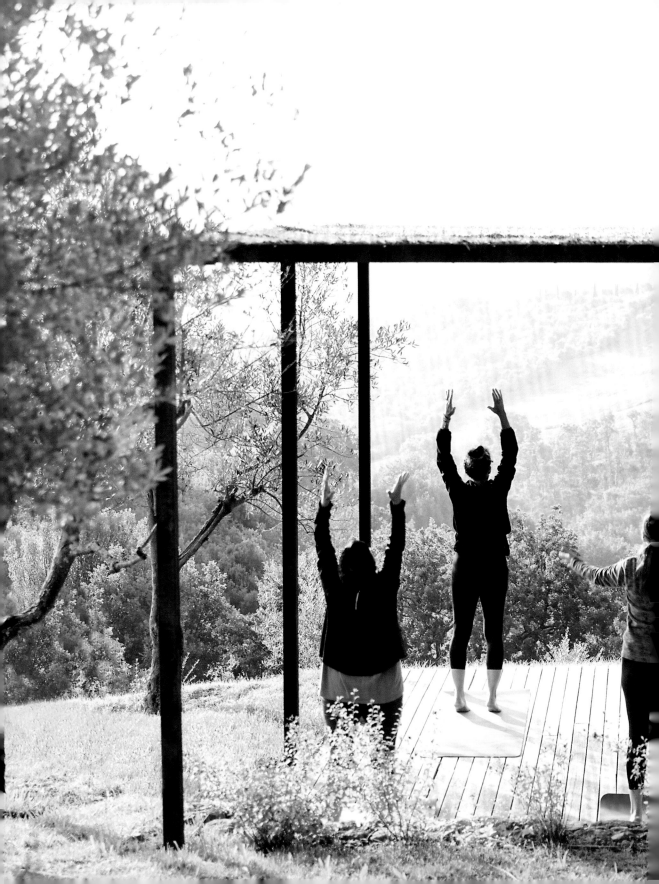

Move the Body, Calm the Mind

A Different Way of Thinking About Exercise

SO MANY OF US HAVE A LOVE-HATE, completely guilt-ridden relationship with exercise. That is definitely me. Though I have never been a big fan of the gym, I have tried every fitness regimen going. When I was modelling in London, I spent hours cheek-to-butt with aerobics fanatics, "feeling the burn." During my hectic TV years, I booked private trainers to come to the house for painfully early morning sessions for both me and Hans. I have to admit that the fights over who would get up and answer the doorbell for the five a.m. session shook even my solid marriage! I once gave Hans a gym membership for his birthday, and he did go off one morning, wearing a pair of his son's tatty school shorts and a T-shirt that he normally wore to bed. He slipped a disc, was carried out on a stretcher and never returned to the gym. I can't blame him when I think of how many gyms I've joined in the new year only to have the membership fizzle by February. Still, I have done so many sit-ups in my time, I reassure myself that deep underneath the layers of flesh (which I blame on my children), I have abs of steel.

I remember chuckling when a guest at Villa Reniella asked me to show him our gym. Confused by my response, he stared blankly in the direction I was pointing: where was the building? The villa sits partway up a steep hill, with barely any flat land around it. To keep fit here, we do not need running machines, elliptical trainers or a barrage of weights. Run or walk up and down these hills, and there is your workout. I spend my days in motion: hiking downhill to check on the pond's water level and to see how the lower olive grove is progressing, then lugging myself

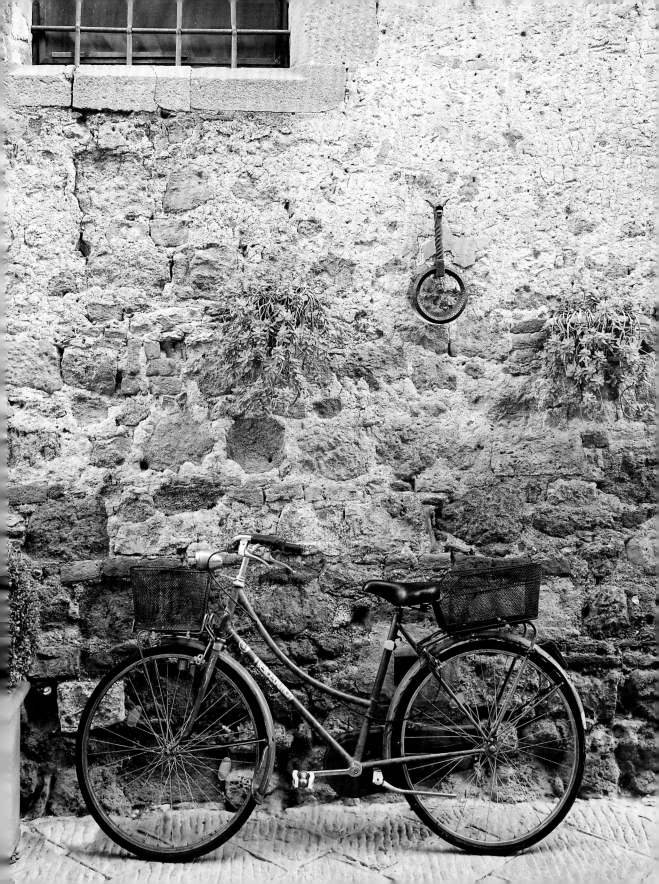

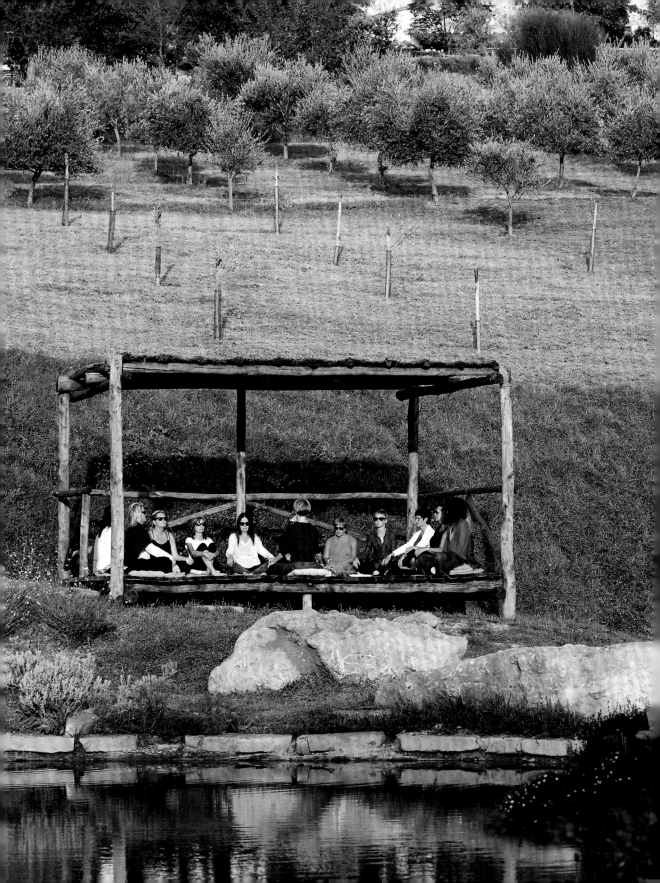

back up to the villa. We do have a yoga platform, with a beautiful view over the valley, but instead of yoga, I'm constantly picking up discarded mats and the odd wineglass and carrying them up to the house. All of us who work at the villa bend and twist our way from dawn to dusk, pulling up the ever-sprouting weeds, picking olives, clipping vines, digging or harvesting in the garden. We always seem to be moving furniture around. Then, at the end of the day, we head up the steep cypress-lined lane to the bar in the piazza for a well-deserved Aperol spritz. This life is not what I ever imagined an exercise routine to be, but these Tuscan hills have me the fittest I have ever been.

Many Italians seem exercise-shy in the North American sense of the word, but their fitness routine revolves around natural movement throughout the day, plenty of walking and using all of the body's muscles. Even the oldest of our neighbours are usually in motion. They mend stuff, stroll around the markets and climb trees to pick olives. They take a daily walk with friends, work their gardens and help others with their chores.

Nearly all of Tuscany's walled medieval towns were built on hilltops, with wide views over the surrounding countryside, so that when the bad guys were marching towards the town, they could be easily spotted. The early warning such locations offered was well worth the challenge to the thighs. Cars (apart from delivery vehicles) are still banned from these settlements, so locals and tourists alike move around by foot. I remember how I huffed and puffed up the stairs of the apartment I rented here during the villa renovation—I was on the fifth floor of a crumbling palazzo with no elevator. I admit I was actually brought to tears each time I realized I'd forgotten something in the car, parked outside the village gates, and had to climb all the way down the stairs and back to get it, then haul whatever it was—a heavy box of sample tiles, for instance—along the steep streets and up the stairs again. A nightmare, as I always seemed to be out of breath and would often find myself alongside a little old lady effortlessly carrying *her* heavy bags. Now I can keep pace!

What I have learned from these village elders about living a vital life well into old age is the importance of daily movement that exercises all the muscles and lubricates all the joints of the body. A one-hour spin class three times a week has its benefits, but it will not balance out the endless hours you spend sitting at a computer or slumped in front of the television. We know from longevity research that the key to living a long, healthy life is balance in all things. Choose a workout you enjoy—a run, a boxing class, Pilates—but keep moving all day long. Stand up from your desk and stretch every thirty minutes, or even better, go for a walk. Take the stairs instead of the elevator. Park the car a ten-minute walk from your destination, wherever you're heading and whatever the weather (within reason, of course). Don't grab the phone and scroll through Instagram while taking a break from work—that can be fun, but your body needs to stretch. Constantly moving around is good for your digestion, heart and brain, as well as your muscles and joints.

The *Passeggiata*

I love this time-honoured Italian tradition, where at roughly the same time every day, between five and eight p.m., everyone goes for a walk. Some may just head over to the bar in the piazza as their version of the *passeggiata*, but most undertake a long promenade before dinner. They may stroll or power walk, alone or arm in arm. An elderly mother walks with her daughter, a couple of teenage boys stroll together, overtaking a line of gossiping women whose little children are running ahead of them. In the city, people often dress up for the walk, showing off the latest fashions even as they engage in this age-old ritual.

Jacky and I often join the locals for their evening stroll. She tells me that the *passeggiata* is not a huge calorie-burner, but it has countless health benefits. As you walk at a decent pace, you take in more air, oxygenating the blood. Walking also helps declutter the mind, strengthens muscle tone and lubricates the joints.

The treasured Italian custom of walking with a friend, a colleague or family at the end of the day is a vital way to socialize *and* move. Add this habit to your routine and I promise you will see the benefits in years to come.

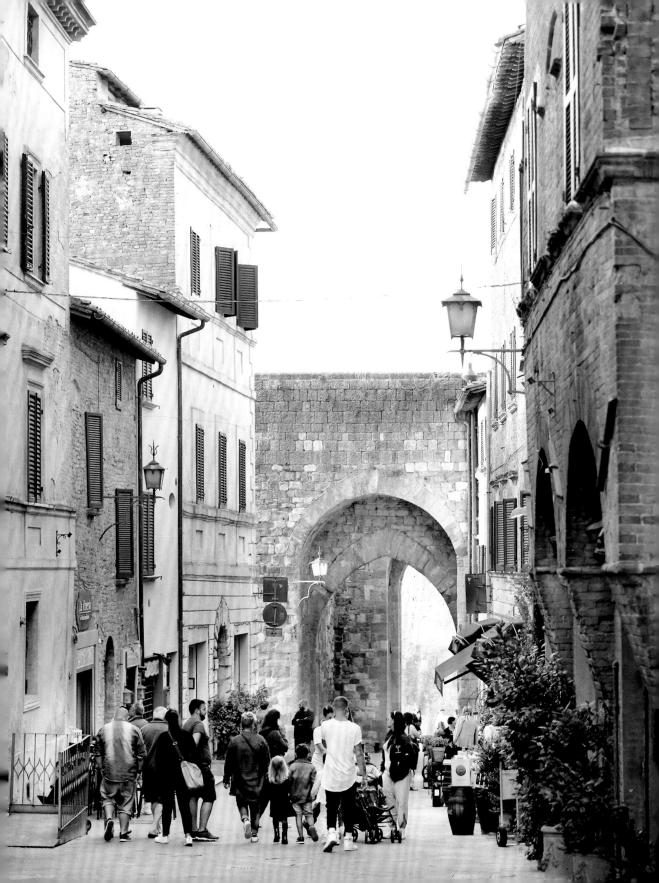

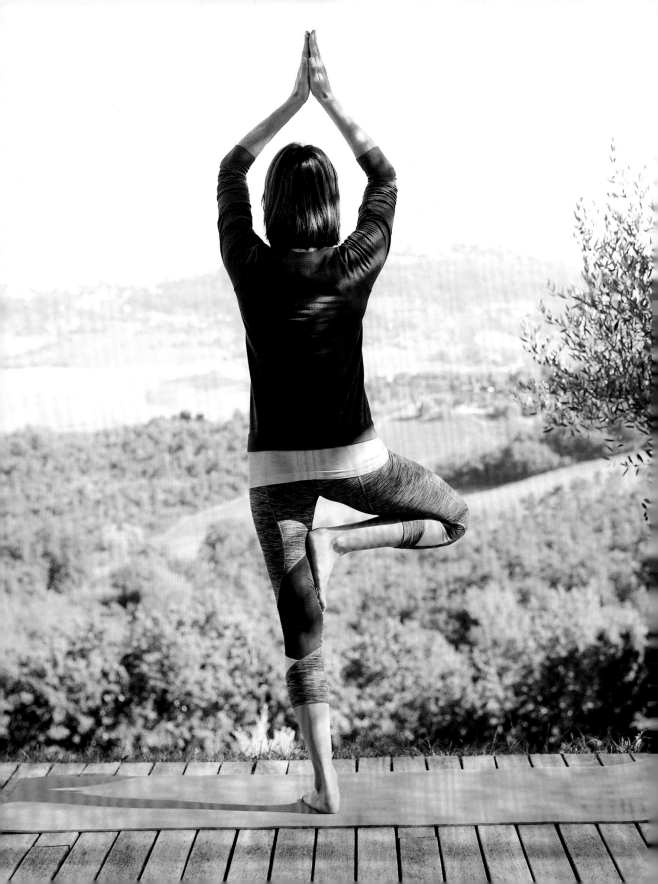

JACKY SAYS

Exercise releases adrenaline, which stimulates the heart to pump blood around the body faster, delivering oxygen to the muscles. The lungs work harder and your rate of respiration increases. Well-oxygenated blood goes to the brain and, immediately, the brain cells start functioning at a higher level, making you feel more alert and focused.

Exercise also triggers the neurotransmitters serotonin, which helps regulate our mood, and dopamine, called the "pleasure" hormone. It releases endorphins, which stimulate a sense of euphoria (you've heard of the "runner's high"?), and glutamate, a neurotransmitter that activates your muscles to keep you moving.

The wonders of regular exercise are immeasurable. It wards off depression, increases energy, helps control weight, helps prevent heart disease, ameliorates the effects of type 2 diabetes and reduces your chances of developing chronic diseases.

Finding the Calm Within Us

As our world becomes increasingly out of balance, we yearn to find the calm within us. For many, the movements and breath work of yoga are the answer, which likely explains why yoga's popularity has grown in parallel with the escalated pace of our daily lives and the stress of the coronavirus lockdowns.

If you haven't tried yoga before, give it a whirl. Remember, there isn't just one style of yoga; there are many types of practices with different focuses: spiritual, bodily, energy-releasing and meditative. If one teacher doesn't suit you, search until you find one that meets your needs. But don't base your decision solely on your comfort! Yoga practice should also be challenging. Years ago, Jacky and I joined a yoga "chair" class, which was exactly as described. After getting constantly tangled between the legs and the back of an institutional metal chair and finally tipping over, chin first, I never returned. Jacky loved it.

At the Tuscan getaways, we bless the awakening of each new day with yoga. The point of the early-morning ritual is not the bending, stretching and wrapping one's limbs into a pretzel shape, but the camaraderie. The dawn chorus of women chirping away as they wander down to the yoga platform is heaven to me—some are a little dubious, if it's their first time, but the rest are blissfully ready to stretch.

If yoga really isn't your thing, there are other Eastern approaches you can try that work the body and still the mind. For years I've been mesmerized by the sunrise goings-on in a park on the edge of Chinatown, near my place in Toronto, where a group gathers to practise the serene rhythmic flow of qigong—apparently unaware of the intrusive traffic, the dog walkers and the likes of myself watching them from the sidelines. They seem lost in another world. Qigong refers to the life energy, qi, that streams through the pathways of the body. Its Chinese masters say: "Movement is the consequence of qi (energy force). Qi follows intention. Intention is directed with the mind."

I tried a qigong class on a trip to Thailand. It's difficult to let your thoughts drift towards the to-do lists of the day when you need to coordinate your posture, movement and breathing all at the same time, without toppling over. After a session, energy flows through the body and sharpens the mind like a shot of espresso. I was hooked. I practise for twenty minutes at the start of each day, alone in my pyjamas because none of the Tuscan locals partake in this very foreign ritual. I have been tempted to do my qigong one morning in the village piazza, if only to see the bemused looks on their faces. I very much doubt anyone will join me.

Settle Down and Breathe—Deeply!

Jacky and I once attended a class on a breathing technique called pranayama where I thought I was going to die laughing. I didn't dare look at her for fear I'd crack right up and we'd both be ejected. I just couldn't get over the fact that all the serious yogis we were sitting cross-legged among were blowing their noses into thin air and panting with extended tongues. This type of deep breath work is supposed to instantly settle the mind, but instead I was riveted to the nose of a rather large, sweaty gentleman, who was surrounded by wet tissues as he blew giant bubbles from each nostril in turn.

Many different breathing techniques have been practised for their calming and centring effects for thousands of years, but I had a hard time finding one. Take lion's pose, or simhasana, where you kneel on all fours, then stick your tongue out as far

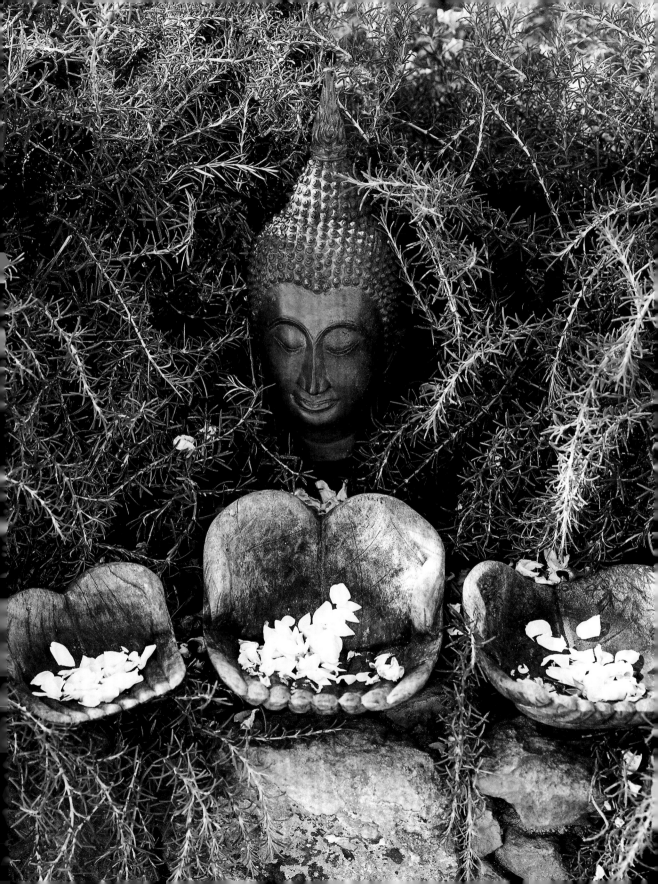

as possible and roar. More helpless laughter. Feeling useless, I gave up on breathing for awhile (not *all* breathing, of course). Then my son—the one who works for an international non-governmental organization—was posted to another war-torn country, where the situation was still extremely volatile, terrifying his parents. The villa's yoga instructor, Rupert, told me I needed to breathe and managed to teach me a technique that worked.

Maybe your mother told you to count to ten when you were having a meltdown as a child—and it worked! It wasn't the counting that calmed you down, but taking your mind off the incident. Deep breathing, by whatever technique, calms a person's agitation and defuses anger. A breathing session, either in a group or alone at the end of the day, is a simple way to de-stress. Add a few minutes of conscious breathing to your day: count to five in your head as you breathe in and count to five in your mind as you breathe out. Repeat. You can do this anywhere: on the bus to work, while stuck in traffic or even standing in line at the supermarket. (In the age of COVID-19, though, maybe practise these techniques at home or at a safe distance from others.)

By mindfully taking deliberate deep breaths, it is possible to stimulate the vagus nerve—the longest nerve in the body, running from the brain and wandering around the major organs to the gut—slowing down your heartbeat and lowering stress.

Seek Inner Peace

Much of what I've learned in Tuscany is about the importance of community, close friends and gathering together. But there are times when the best thing we can do for ourselves is to be alone.

The villa is often a noisy place. There is always something going on. When a group of women get together, the conversations have few limits, and while they can be beautiful and inspiring, they are never quiet. I admit that most evenings during retreats, I wander off in search of a few minutes of solitude. We all need a place to sit quietly with our own thoughts—or no thoughts at all. My favourite spot is a small overgrown field just down the hill from the villa and guest rooms; it is such

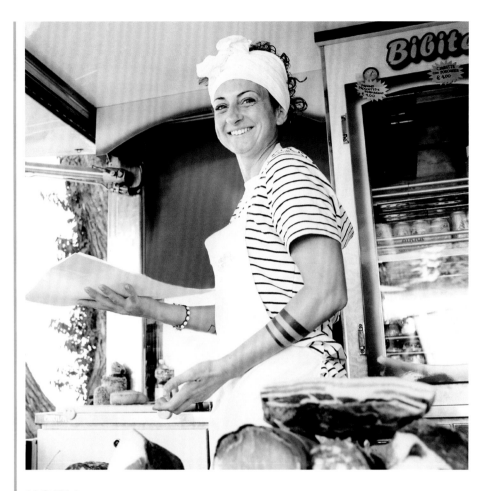

MONIA

Monia is the embodiment of the super-busy, modern woman. Her family's prosciutto business is legendary in these parts; she spends her days behind the counter serving slices of cured meat and traditional porchetta sandwiches, and juggling the demands of her large family. Her solace and respite is painting. She tries to steal a break from the hurly-burly of her life every day, making a mad dash for the tiny painting studio behind her home. "Before I pick up my brush," she says, "I close my eyes and empty my mind for ten minutes. It is remarkable how a short meditation becomes the bridge between two different worlds, allowing me to feel grounded and still. By calming myself right down, I am flooded with creativity and I'm ready to paint."

a magical place, we eventually dug a big hole for a pond, which we surrounded with aquatic plants, then built a pergola that floats above it. Though I still visit on my own to watch the Tuscan sunset, members of our retreat groups now come here to meditate. And so do I.

At first, I admit, I felt silly, sitting on the meditation platform with my eyes closed and my back straight, trying desperately to calm my mind. But with practice, I've become dedicated to the positive feelings—gratitude, joy and contentment— that emerge when I take this precious time to still myself. Pam, the mindfulness therapist who works with us at the villa, doesn't ask us to try to empty our minds, but simply to sit, in silence and stillness, in this secluded place with the endless view. Gradually, we become aware of the flow of our thoughts and feelings, as the busyness of the day drops away. When, as Pam teaches, I can just observe my thoughts and feelings without getting caught up in them, I feel my mind growing more spacious at the same time as I sink into the physical world centred on my body and my breathing.

Meditation is similar to praying, whatever the religion. It is a practice of being present in the moment in order to find a place from which you can view your own struggles with kindness and compassion. You need to be patient with yourself when you're learning to meditate. At first, your thoughts will constantly wander to your to-do list, or what's for dinner, or what you should pack for an upcoming trip. But then you will notice how you feel after each short session, and eventually you will become eager to use this tool frequently to improve your mental and physical well-being. Regular meditation can help reduce emotional volatility, enhance the body's immune function and improve concentration. It also promotes a healthier perspective when we are dealing with conflict, crisis or loss in our lives.

Many of the residents of the small Tuscan villages around us have never jour- neyed beyond Rome or Florence, let alone to another country. Their lives are simple, attuned to the daily rhythms of work, sustenance and family. They don't seem to be in a perpetual search for something they don't already have. Can we learn from them? The guests at our villa come from all walks of life, and each has their own reason for being here. Some visit to experience the beauty of this corner of the world, some come longing to meet like-minded others, and most just want to have a good time. But they all bring their own life stories, which can include a measure of pain and loss, and they all participate with trepidation and then pure delight in the meditation workshop.

Mindfulness and meditation invite us to pause from our constant struggle to improve ourselves and others, and appreciate our lives, not as we think they *should* be, but just as they are. And once we've taken that measure of ourselves, we can find the space to ask how essential all the things are with which we fill our days. Do we really need to rush from one activity to another? Is it possible that we might be better off with less? Pam has seen mindfulness transform many lives.

I view our mediation sessions as a lasting gift to our guests. Once you've learned how to meditate, you can take that knowledge with you wherever you go, through the good times and the bad. When the retreat is over and everyone returns home, I'm hopeful that something of these workshops goes with them. I know for myself the ways in which mindfulness cultivates our capacity to respond skilfully to whatever life throws at us.

How to Bring Tuscany Home

- Take a tip from our ancestors, who never sat at a desk all day. Keep moving!
- Nudge yourself to get up from your desk or chair and stretch and walk around every thirty minutes.
- Park a ten-minute walk from your destination and travel the rest of the way by foot.
- Create your own *passeggiata*. Take a stroll as often as you can with a friend, your family or a walking group.
- Declutter your mind with regular meditation. Even five minutes a day will make a difference.
- Remember to breathe deeply! It will help you control challenging situations.
- Try yoga, tai chi, qigong or any other practice that gently moves every part of your body.
- Find a type of exercise that gives you pleasure as it raises your heartbeat and stretches and strengthens your muscles. If exercise feels good, you will stick to it.
- Take the time to observe how you feel after exercise, deep breathing and meditation; you'll want to do more!

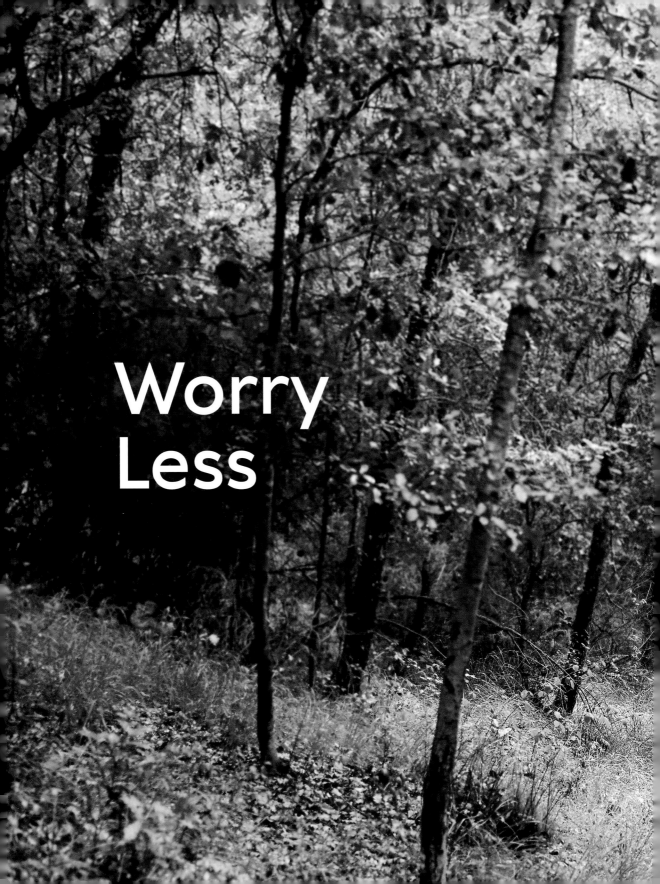

Worry
Less

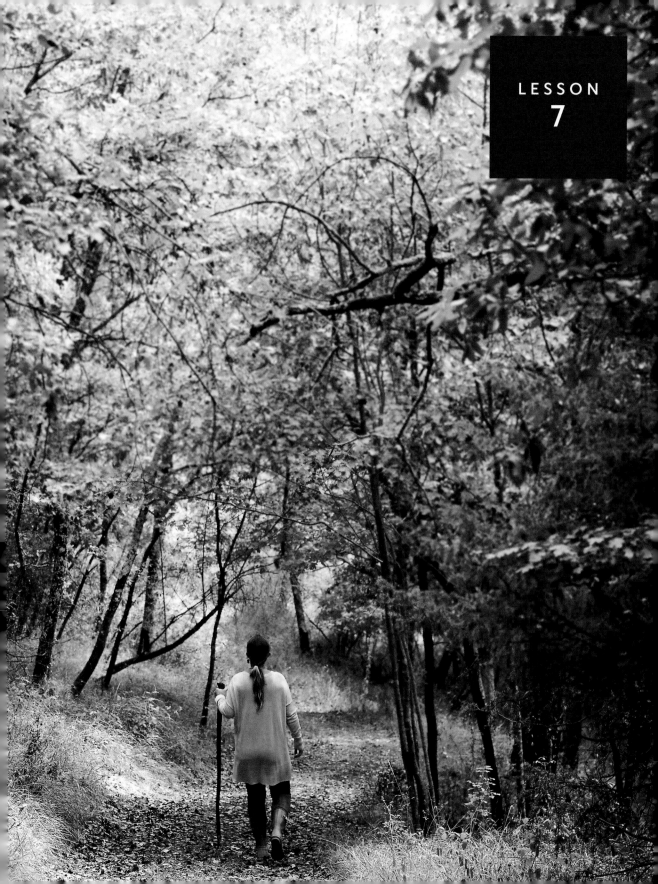

LESSON
7

No Word in Italian for Stress

REALLY, THERE IS NO DIRECT ITALIAN TRANSLATION of the word *stress*. But that doesn't mean people in Italy are never stressed. I've never met anyone here who insists their life is the *dolce vita* tourists tend to imagine. The country has severe economic problems, which weren't made any better by the pandemic, its government rarely runs smoothly, and it's dealing with tensions caused by a constant stream of refugees crossing the Mediterranean from Africa.

But, and it is a big but, Italy's people, especially in rural areas, have evolved many ways of handling day-to-day problems that keep stress and anxiety in perspective. There's much we can learn from how these neighbours of mine express and deal with the friction of life—lessons that can be incorporated into our own hectic worlds.

First, let's get our terms straight. *Stress* is the immediate reaction to a specific situation, whereas *anxiety* is a continuous worried feeling that's hard to shake and doesn't seem to have a specific trigger. That knot in the stomach, the sense that disaster is about to strike. The endless "what ifs." When we're in an anxious state, something we hear on the news can send us into a spiral, even if it has nothing directly to do with us. A troubling phone call has us reaching for the wine bottle; we can't face the lineup of meetings or chores we face each day; and we wake up in the morning with a sense of dread rather than excitement.

In most countries today, stress and anxiety levels are soaring, a crisis caused by the pandemonium of our everyday lives. The World Health Organization has called stress "the health epidemic of the twenty-first century" and describes burnout as an

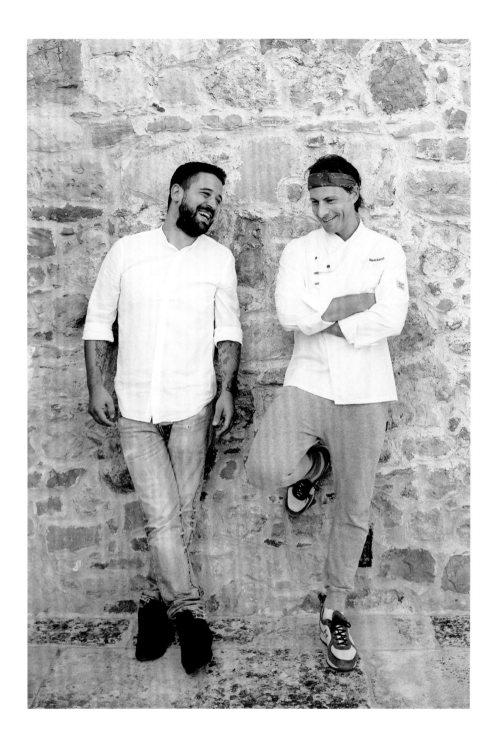

WORRY LESS

"occupational phenomenon." The assaults on our equilibrium can be as mundane as losing the car keys, as catastrophic as losing a partner and as bewildering and frightening as a new virus striking our world. Our anxiety and stress can become so pervasive that they even stress out the people around us. Really coming to grips with this health crisis will require efforts by governments and businesses. It's not all down to us as individuals to find a path away from anxiety, but there are many things we can do that will help, as my Italian friends have taught me.

Restless nights, low energy, irritability, loss of desire, headaches, aches and pains, and even a rapid heartbeat are all signs of stress and anxiety. How can we find joy when we are drowning in worry? We often try to cope in ways that provide some immediate relief but have long-term negative consequences. We gulp down ready-made food that's low in nutrition, drink too much, smoke another cigarette, take drugs (and I don't mean prescribed anti-anxiety medications, which some people truly need), lose ourselves in social media and lash out at the people around us. Gosh, I am stressed just writing this.

I am often asked if my decision to move to a rural community in the middle of Italy has lowered my stress levels. The answer is yes and no. I'm pinch-myself happy here in my valley, but my life is not all roses. Still, the daily problems I face feel way more manageable than those I encountered rushing from meeting to meeting in the city and worrying about whether a television series would be cancelled and the entire team would lose their jobs; the pressure was immense. Here, I get completely frantic when a guest comes flying off her bike headfirst into a ditch and has to be rushed to hospital (yes, it happened, and thank heavens she was fine). And it's also panic stations if the pond we dug in my favourite spot springs a leak in its liner and, for the thirtieth time, the town water board cuts me off. Recently, a member of Germany's former royal family joined a car rally event we were hosting here. Within minutes of checking in, he turned up in the kitchen to announce that there was a leg hanging through his bedroom ceiling. Thankfully, it turned out to still be attached to the plumber, who'd been checking a pipe on the roof and had gone through a faulty tile. I wasn't sure of the royal protocol: should I laugh, cry or rip my hair out?

I have learned a great deal from the Italian response to life's vicissitudes, and that knowledge is at the core of our retreats. Our guests journey to the villa to relax and recharge in breathtaking surroundings. They're so excited to arrive, at first you can't tell their level of burnout or stress. But by the second day, in sympathetic company far away from their everyday lives, their stories tumble forth. Rather than withdrawing in the face of others' distress and their own, the women really connect, acknowledging what they and the others are feeling, showing each other genuine heart. It all comes out: work stress, health problems, child issues, taking care of elderly parents, loneliness, loss of purpose, the heartbreak of death and divorce.

By the end of the week, they are transformed. Jacky and I have shed many a happy tear during these extraordinary last nights, overwhelmed by the difference a week at the villa has made to these beaming women engaged in animated conversation. We are not therapists—far from it. But we have immersed our guests in Tuscan life, and it has had an impact. Their job is to take this mood home and keep the flame burning. And that's the job of this book, too!

Get It Off Your Chest

Sounds crazy, but I do believe that letting loose with a good rant can lower anxiety levels. I remember my mother—who, after she was widowed, had so many challenges in her life, including keeping us all fed—leaning on the rickety back fence, a steaming mug of tea in her hand, chatting to her neighbour about the problems in their small cosmos. She would always return indoors in a better mood. "Right then, back to the ironing," she'd say. "You kids, get on with your homework."

Complaining is a way of life for Italians. Ask a villager how he's feeling and he will probably reply, "Well, I am not dead yet, but . . ." Having come from an overly positive world where we all pretend to be just fine, even fabulous, all the time, I found this hard to get used to. Italians will grumble while drinking with friends, bellyache on a beach as they tuck into a gelato, and moan in the bar while reading the daily news to whoever will listen. Minutes later, they are laughing and cheering each other on, life's tribulations forgotten for now. So often we keep our problems to ourselves, worried about being a burden to our family and friends, but what that attitude does is cut us off from them when we need them most.

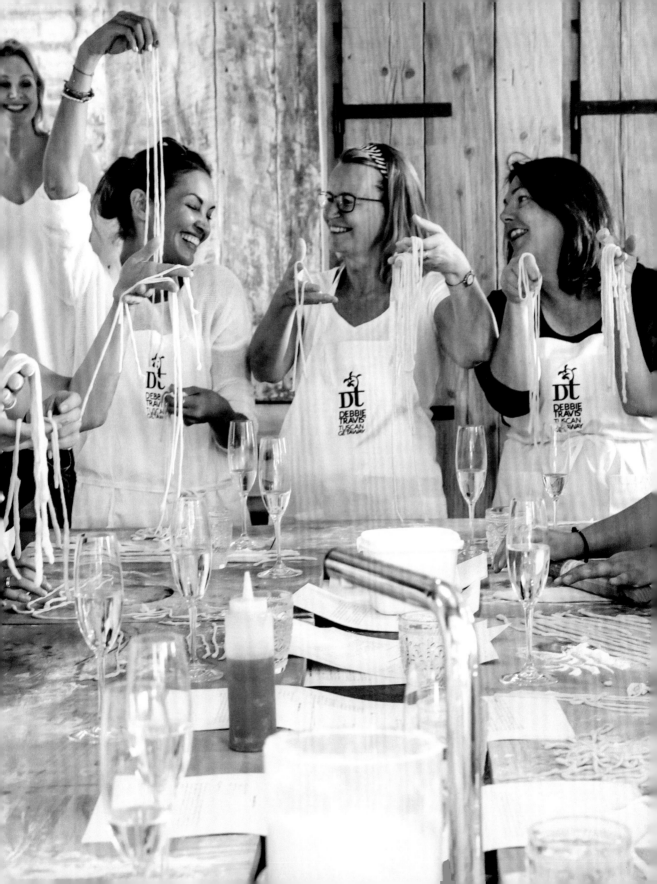

Cook Together

In the warmth of the summer months, in every corner of Italy, gangs of *nonnas* can be found set up on rickety wooden tables in alleyways, kneading pasta. During the cooler days, the ground-floor shutters of the houses are often flung open, allowing us a peek into cluttered kitchens where families are cooking together. The family meal is a religion in the Italian culture, but working together to prepare it is also a natural stress reliever.

From the windows of the fifth-floor apartment I rented while the renovations were going on, tucked under the palazzo's eaves, I could see through the windows of several homes. It was fascinating to watch the early mornings and evenings unfurl in other people's lives. One very old lady, who lived a stone's throw away, seemed to be cooking every time I glanced her way. But at around six each night, another woman, who I assumed was her daughter, would come by to help her for an hour, chatting away as they worked. One day I recognized the younger of the two in the grocery store and introduced myself. I told her how kind I thought she was to visit her mother so often. She said the old lady was actually her neighbour, and that *she* was the one who benefitted most from the visit. She was a lawyer, and every night, on the way home from work, she brought her blood pressure down by spending an hour hanging out with this retiree, chopping vegetables.

One of the highlights of our retreat week is the cooking class. Chef Francesco teaches the group some of the dishes involved in a traditional Tuscan Sunday lunch, which includes preparing pasta from scratch. Chaos reigns in the kitchen, but the camaraderie has a profound effect on everyone. By the time their sleeves are rolled up and they are into the rhythm of kneading the dough, then rolling it out and carefully cutting it into strips, twisting and pinching each piece, any residual anxiety has left the room. I remember one woman exclaiming, "If only I could bottle this feeling I have right now!"

You can. Invite a pal or two around for a Sunday afternoon pasta-making extravaganza. It costs nothing except the price of some flour, eggs and oil. Make a lovely mess as you cook together and then gobble up the fruits of your labour. The warmth you will feel is the catalyst to do it again and again. It is hard to be anxious when you're having so much fun.

PICI AL FUMO

Pici is a thick, homemade Tuscan pasta with deep peasant roots. It resembles a larger, fatter spaghetti and, when cooked, it is the perfect size and texture to hold a robust sauce. Pici al fumo is a dish that comes from Chef Francesco's hometown of Cortona, which is also where *Under the Tuscan Sun* was filmed. The "fumo" refers to the smokiness created by the bacon in the rose-coloured sauce.

PICI:

3 cups flour, plus more for sprinkling and as needed

1 egg

Big pinch of salt

1 tablespoon extra virgin olive oil

TOMATO AND SMOKED BACON SAUCE:

3 tablespoons extra virgin olive oil

1 onion, chopped

1½ cups finely diced smoked bacon or pancetta

2 cups plain tomato sauce (from a jar or homemade)

1 cup light cream

A few fresh sage and rosemary leaves

Salt and freshly ground pepper

TO SERVE:

Finely grated pecorino or Parmesan cheese

To make the pici: On a clean, flat surface, pile the flour in a small mound and make a well in the centre. Crack the egg into the well, then add the salt. Mix the egg gently with a fork. Add the olive oil to the well, then flour your hands and begin mixing it all together, incorporating the flour little by little into the egg and oil. Once it's combined, move the dough onto a floured surface and knead for about 10 minutes, until it becomes smooth and compact. If it feels sticky, add flour a teaspoon at a time until the dough smooths out. If it's a little stiff and dry, add cold water a teaspoon at a time until it's moist and pliable.

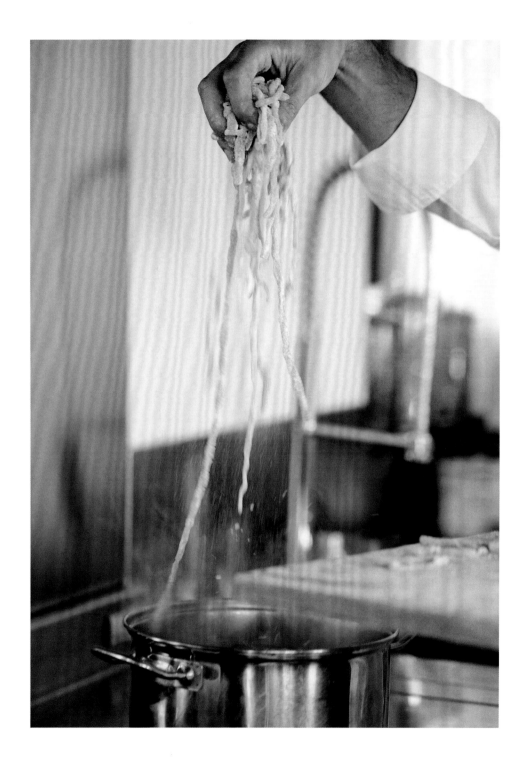

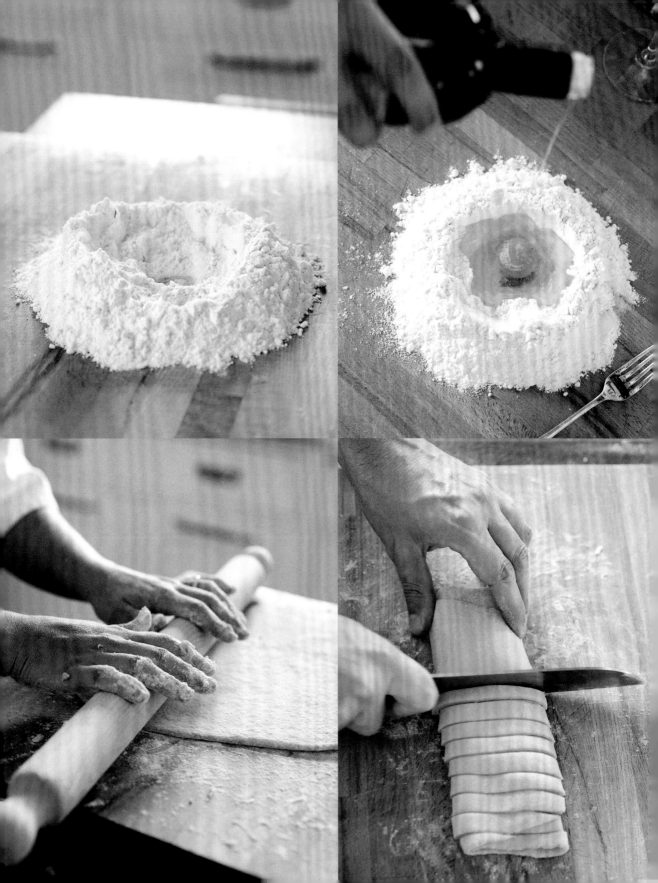

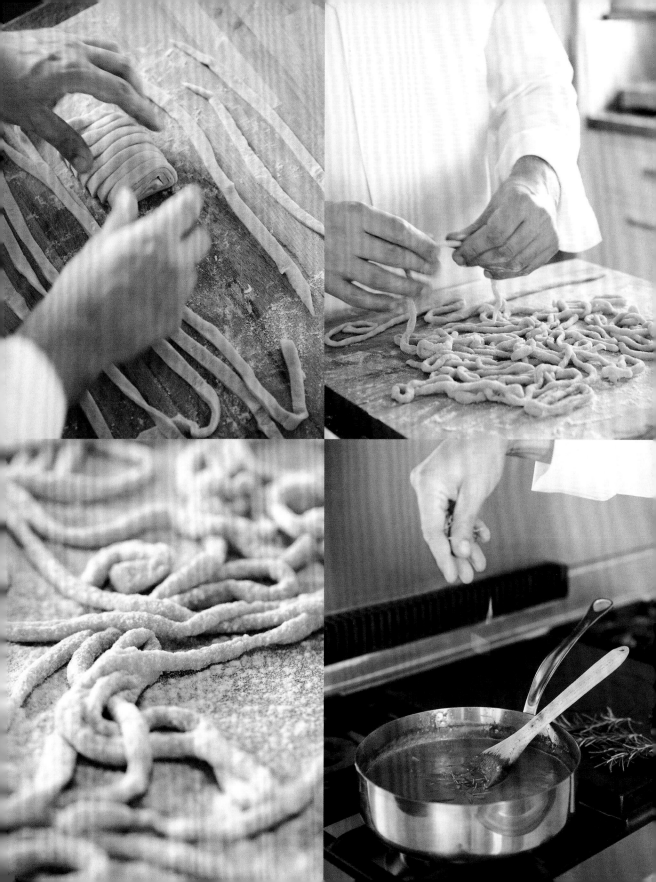

You can use a pasta machine, but it's more fun to hand-roll the dough. Get out your longest rolling pin and roll the dough into a sheet roughly $\frac{1}{16}$ inch (2 mm) thick. Lightly flour the pasta and fold, sprinkling a little more flour on the unfloured surfaces as you fold so it won't stick together. Cut the pasta into strips about the same width as a tagliatelle noodle (about ¾ inch/1.5 cm). Keep the strands from sticking together with more sprinkles of flour. Using your thumbs and forefingers, roll, twist and press each strand of pasta until it becomes the irregular hand-rolled shape of Tuscan pici. Set the pasta aside.

To make the sauce: In a frying pan, heat the olive oil over medium heat. Sauté the onion until translucent. Add the bacon and sauté for a few minutes longer. Once the bacon and onions have had some time to mingle, add the tomato sauce, lower the heat and simmer for another 10 minutes. Add the cream, sage and rosemary, and simmer for 10 more minutes, careful not to let the sauce boil. Season to taste with salt and pepper.

To cook the pasta: Meanwhile, bring a pot of salted water to a boil over high heat. Add the pici and boil for 5 minutes or until al dente. (Check by taking a noodle out and cutting it to see if it is nearly cooked through. You'll know it's perfect when you see a very small speck of uncooked dough in the middle of the noodle. If there is more than a speck, the pasta needs more time.)

To serve: Drain the cooked pasta, then pour it into a big bowl. Add the sauce and stir until coated. Serve with pecorino or Parmesan.

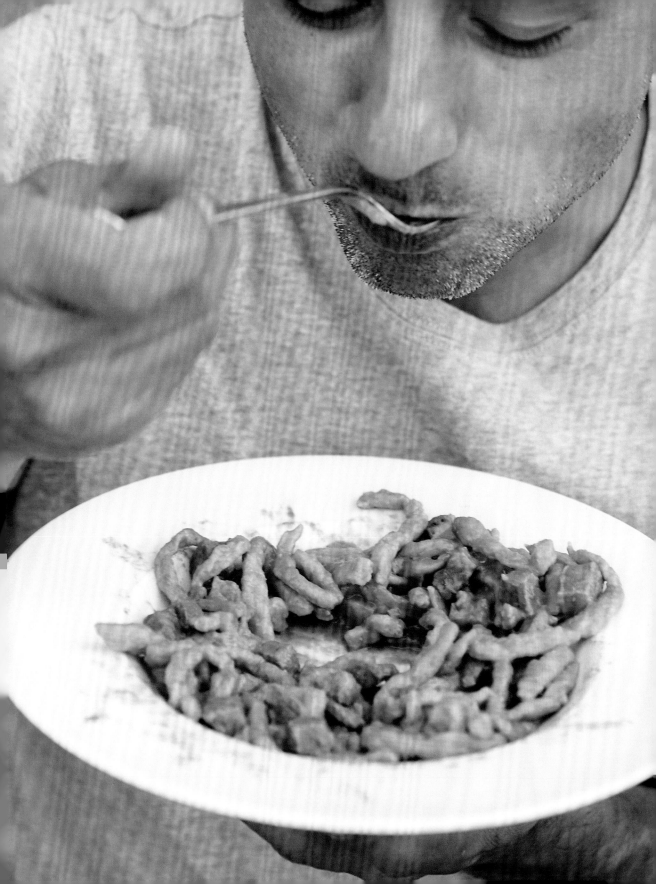

Forest Bathing

Not a day goes by when I'm at home in Tuscany that I do not walk through the surrounding woods. In these strange times of uncertainty, when the pressure from living through the pandemic often finds me weepy, immersing myself in the trees is the very best medicine. I am never alone. I always encounter an octogenarian foraging for a mysterious herb or a dog walker out for a stroll, all of us finding peace of mind.

It is the same the world over: we are all drawn to nature, and for good reason. Research has shown that time spent under nature's canopy is critical to fighting depression and stress, and has other health benefits, too. A walk in the woods activates areas of the brain called the default mode network, which come to life when we break away from our daily routine of chores and work and commuting. How many light bulbs have gone off for you when you've been gardening, lying in savasana pose or even standing in the shower? A walk in the woods, in particular, both calms us and releases our creativity. Make a daily walk a priority. Even if you can't get to the woods, simply walking and looking at the world around you will set your mind free.

The Five-by-Five Rule, Tuscan Style

Oh, how I wish I had known and obeyed this rule while I was raising two active boys and running my television productions. I am an impulsive person. ("No kidding!" I can hear my friends and colleagues saying.) In the old days, when my stress escalated, I could put a karate fighter to shame with my knee-jerk reactions. I once came home, tired and filthy, from a busy day filming and renovating. Washing off the first layer of grime at the kitchen sink, I smelled what I thought was marijuana smoke slinking in the window from the backyard, where I could see my fourteen-year-old standing. Without a moment's thought, I yelled, "Are you smoking dope! Get inside and go to your bedroom. You're grounded!" I was just calling his dad when my lad came into the kitchen and calmly said, "I was burning the leaves like Dad told me to." He *was* burning leaves, I realized, when I calmed down enough to actually look out into the backyard. If I'd only deployed the five-by-five rule before I blew up, I wouldn't have been flooded with guilt for the rest of the night, and I would not still be the butt of my son's teasing all these years later.

The rule is simple. Before reacting to a stressful situation, take a moment to ask whether it will matter in five minutes, five days or five years. If the answer is no, it's like magic: your stress evaporates and you can flip the negative energy of the situation into a positive and find a solution. This is so typically Italian. "*Piano, piano,*" they say (still pretty often to me). *Slowly, slowly,* let's just work this out.

And here's a perfect example of their attitude at work. At the retreats, we take our guests out for several meals in nearby restaurants. I book the tables months in advance, since many of them are small spaces and they need lots of notice to arrange a table for twenty. I always triple-check the date and the time, but I knew that sooner or later we were bound to run into a problem. When we did, it was a Sunday lunchtime in summer, when it seems like every Italian family, along with the deluge of tourists, is packed into pizza joints, trattorias and restaurants. The particular place I'd chosen has a stunning view of rolling hills carpeted in golden wheat fields; the prime seating is on the terrace. And here was the head waiter telling me when I turned up at the door, "Oops, was it this week?" Luckily, the women were too busy tumbling out of the vans and staring around at the picturesque town to take in my panicked face as visions of a ham sandwich picnic for twenty raced through my mind.

It could have gone two ways. If I'd lost my temper, we would have been into the blame game, with me shouting, "How could this happen? I checked three times! We will never come back here again!" All my bridges to a lovely restaurant would have been burned, and I would have created an ugly scene for the staff and the people trying to enjoy their lunch. Instead, I breathed deeply and explained my situation. The head waiter and the restaurant staff launched into a flurry of incomprehensible Italian, arms waving. I wasn't sure what was happening until I saw the chef and several waiters running towards me down the ancient cobbled street, carrying folding tables and a variety of mismatched chairs. I grinned in relief, but then turned to stare at the already full patio. Where would they put twenty more people?

Only in Italy, I thought, as the staff asked the other patrons to stand, pasta dangling from their forks, and move, then sit again, way more squished together. No one was upset! Instead, as everyone crammed in, new friendships were made and wine on the house was offered all around. I waved a thank you to the head waiter, who hollered over the customers' heads, "*Non c'est problema, fa niente*"— "Don't worry about it, it's nothing." The Tuscan mantra: go with the flow, there are worse things that can happen, let's find a solution. I wonder if the waiter had ever heard of the five-by-five rule.

To Thine Own Self Be True

Understanding yourself is the key to lowering your anxiety levels. Can you identify what's driving your stress? Sometimes, simple questions can show you the way. Why do you say yes to stuff you know you don't really want to take on? Why do you think you can or even should squeeze something else into an already overstuffed day, given that at the end of it, you'll feel like you didn't pay enough attention to anything? Do you simply find it easier to give in to other people's demands than to find your own path?

Take a good look at your daily schedule. Is it all just too much? Once we are honest with ourselves about what's stressing us out and keeping us that way, we can begin to accept our limitations and find more time for what is really important. We often believe that worrying can somehow solve our problems, when actually we spend too much time caught in a cycle of worrying to actually tackle the issue that's bothering us. With strategic thinking, we can break our worries down into small, manageable, fixable bites.

The Tuscans, traditionally farmers, have spent centuries obeying the weather and the seasons, planting when they need to, harvesting when they must, and eating and sleeping well so they are up for the rigours and demands of such a life. But all Italians seem just as in love with routine as my agricultural neighbours, with their espressos at the café every morning and their lunch breaks that begin at one o'clock sharp. There's a comfort in knowing what's ahead each day, and the order in which it will come, that Italians seem to find essential to living. I've never yet heard an Italian going on and on about how busy and overworked they are. Instead, they tell me about their marvellous naps, yummy lunches and time spent chatting with neighbours and family.

We follow their lead at the villa. We do have a routine, but our motto is *Non Ho Orario*, loosely meaning *I do not have a schedule—there is nothing I have to do!*

I admit the motto came about by accident after I happened upon a job lot of linens on sale when a hotel's deal with an American celebrity fell through; everything from pillowcases to bathrobes was monogrammed with her initials: NHO. The bathrobes were not only gorgeous but were such a bargain I bought the whole lot. Rather than unpicking all the monograms, I decided the initials would inspire our Italian motto (though one guest suggested it should stand for *No Hang Over—* brilliant).

From the moment the retreaters arrive until they head for the airport, they don't have to spend a moment thinking about their schedules, because we've got it covered. The result is that they can let themselves fully relax into the moment. We design each day to keep stress levels low and happiness high. It works like a dream (usually).

I know no one can run their life like it's a non-stop retreat at the villa, but we *can* aim for less stress and more joy.

The Power of Friendship

Most evenings you will find three very old women sitting on a low wall in the village piazza, feet dangling, watching the world go by. They speak occasionally to each other, but they are such old friends that much of what there is to say between them has already been said. Yet even a stranger passing by can see the comfort they find in each other's company.

Friendships, new and old, are the most important element in relieving life's pain and stress. I'm best friends with my husband and my sons, but it's Jacky Brown, my pal of thirty-five years, who is my sister in more ways than I can ever explain, even to her.

I think of my friends, dotted around the globe, as a strand of pearls, each one individual in its beauty, flaws and all. I have collected them over the years, and I cherish them, finding them crucial to my happiness and sanity. The big moves I've made in my life have tested my ability to hang on to my friends. At sixteen, I left the confines of a rural village in the North of England for the eye-opening streets of London, knowing nobody. At twenty-eight, I met a man and minutes after saying "I do" moved to Canada, again not knowing a soul. Two decades later, I arrived in Tuscany, where at first, apart from visits from the family, I was alone. In each place I chose to go, I made a substantial effort to build a tribe, because creating friend-ships is as important to me as breathing.

One of my goals is to ensure that all of the retreat's guests go home with a bounty of new buddies, and feel inspired to rekindle old friendships and nourish the ones they hold dear. Long before running my own girls' getaways was even a glim-mer in the back of my mind, I remember visiting my first retreat-style spa, Rancho La Puerta, at the base of Mount Kuchumaa in Mexico, not far from the American border. I arrived alone, a burned-out, wrung-out, teary mess. I immediately loved everything about the place, but what intrigued me most were the communal dining tables. Solo guests like myself were lured out of our private angst and were soon chatting away with strangers, many of whom would become future friends.

I loved my new companions, but my eyes were constantly drawn to the table where a large group of Black women in their fifties sat at mealtimes, deep in conver-sation, sometimes roaring with laughter and sometimes sharing tears. Remember how much I value curiosity? One night, I finally ventured over and asked, "Who *are* you guys?" Patting the seat beside her, one of the women asked me to join them. It turned out they had all met at college in the United States, and even though they now lived all over the place, they had stayed solid friends ever since. They put it down to their determination to spend a week together every year, no matter what. When I asked how they managed that, they burst into laughter. Basically, no one was allowed an excuse to skip out. Not a child's piano recital, or a divorce, or the loss of a job, or sending the kids off to college. "Only death," one of them hooted, "and it better be your own." This was their twenty-fifth reunion.

ESTERINA

Meet Esterina, the beloved owner and matriarch of our local joint. From sunrise to sunset, you will find her scooting from table to table with trays of food and drink, but you'll also notice how often she stops and becomes immersed in a deep discussion with a customer. "I am both priest and life coach," she says with a chuckle. "For many, the bar is their church, a place to unload worries and share gossip." A habit that is part of the DNA of Italy, the daily visit to the bar offers structure and order, which in itself is a stress reducer. "I feel immensely privileged to hear their confessions, and you would not believe what I have heard over the years." She laughs. I can only imagine.

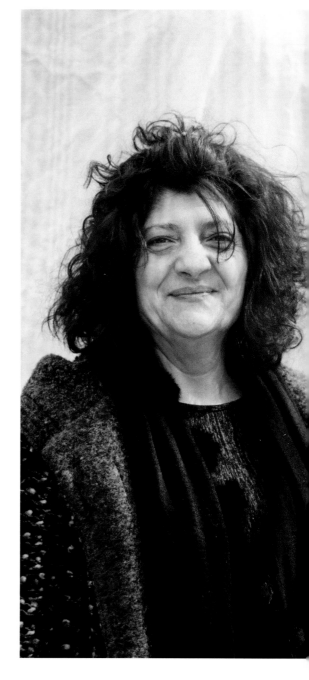

Some of these women were highly groomed and some as casual as it gets. Some clearly had drawn the long straw in life and some the short. They told me they contributed to a fund so that if one of them couldn't afford the week away, they were able to cover the costs for her—that's how important their bond was to them. Circumstance had taken them in different directions, but once a year they met to share their highs and lows with people they trusted and admired; as the week went on, they could feel all their worries and fears diminishing. "We get it all out on the table," one of them summed up. "We prop up one another, finding solutions and the courage to face our burdens—it is priceless."

Yes, it is priceless, and something we all need.

JACKY SAYS

Chronic anxiety can adversely affect us, leading to mental health disorders and other health problems. Learning to control and live with it is vital. Everyone experiences anxiety at some point; you would have to be made of stone to never worry about a thing. Yet when worry escalates, it can cause panic attacks, leading to heart palpitations, chest pains and dizziness. Anxiety can be the root cause of concentration problems, depression, social withdrawal and a non-stop feeling of not being able to cope. It can disturb our sleep and is often the source of insomnia.

Magnesium is known as nature's relaxation mineral, and taking a magnesium supplement before bed can help you sleep. It's always best to ask a qualified health practitioner for advice on such matters, but I take a teaspoon of magnesium powder in water before dropping off.

Anxiety and stress often show themselves through the gut, not only giving you the feeling of a nervous stomach, but, when the gut is tensed, actually affecting the absorption of nutrients. Doctors also connect irritable bowel syndrome with anxiety and treat it with anti-anxiety medications, among other things. If you know that stress hits you in the gut, you can head off worsening symptoms with regular exercise, by ditching excessive caffeine, by sharing problems with others and with calming practices such as yoga and meditation. Spending time in a serene place, away from the overstimulating hustle and bustle, will activate your parasympathetic nervous system (the rest and digest state), easing anxiety. All of the B vitamins, in food and in supplement form, also help support an overtaxed, overstressed nervous system.

How to Bring Tuscany Home

- To discover your stress triggers, keep a diary in which you note people, places and times that create stress in your life. Also jot down what you ate and drank before and after you became anxious.

- Break all of your worries down into solvable chunks, rather than trying to tackle big problems in one go.

- Work on improving your sleep (check out Lesson 3!).

- Share your problems with others, especially in person.

- Prioritize your friendships—keep your old ones and make new ones.

- Learn how to set boundaries and when to say no. Being too busy all the time is a huge source of stress.

- If you notice a connection between your anxiety and what you eat, try an anti-inflammatory Mediterranean diet and see how you feel.

- Try not to eat on the run. A relaxed atmosphere is good for your spirits and your digestion.

- Remember to move your body! And try yoga and meditation.

- Spend as much time in nature as you can.

Divorce Your Devices

(or at Least Kick Them Out for Awhile)

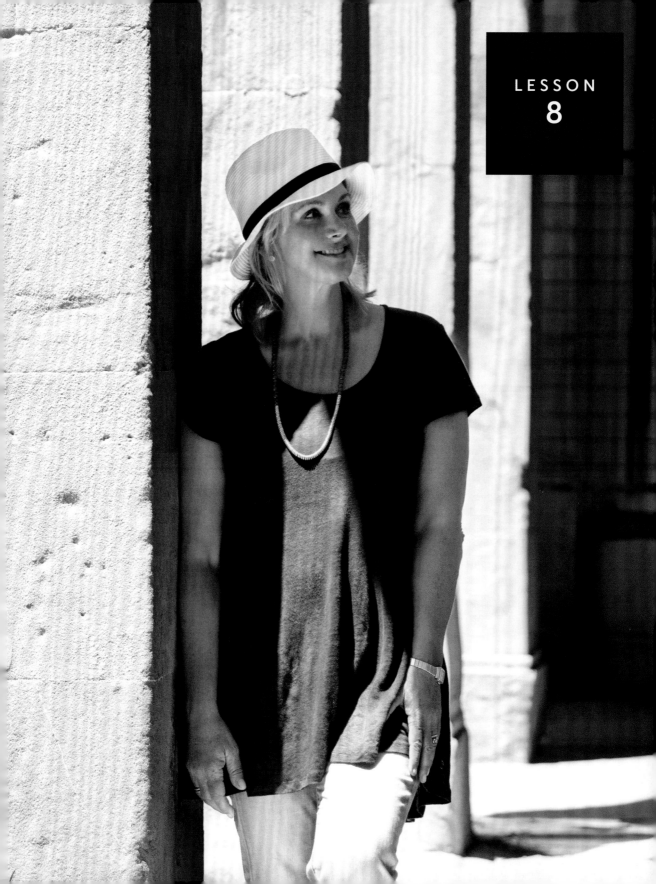

LESSON
8

Screen Time
and Your Brain

ALL ADDICTIONS DISTRACT US FROM LEARNING to be comfortable in our own skin, and we all know how addictive social media and constant texting and messaging can be. During the pandemic, I came to rely on my devices more than ever, as did millions of people locked down at home. Even those of us who used to glare at others who are relentlessly on their phones were deeply thankful for our devices and the Internet and video-calling and streaming apps that kept us connected with our loved ones and our work colleagues.

But enough is enough. To live a joyful, vital life, we need to keep the assault from the digital world in perspective and make sure it doesn't usurp all the other ways we connect as human beings. At the villa, we strongly suggest everyone take a break from technology for the duration of their visit. All of our guests embrace that suggestion, some even telling us that the best part of their week has been "putting that thing away."

I'm from a generation where I remember having to walk to a phone booth to make a call. Then my mum was able to afford a phone, but only one attached to the party line we shared with our neighbours. A teenager's purgatory. My kids grew up with a land line and phones in several rooms in the house; today, the little ones seem to view tablets as an extension of their bodies. We're not about to go backwards when it comes to our connectedness. Like everyone else, in every corner of the world, I cannot live without my cellphone.

The figures are changing by the minute, but as I write this, the average person spends three hours a day on their devices, texting, e-mailing, video-calling, streaming, playing games, taking pictures, browsing Twitter, Instagram and other

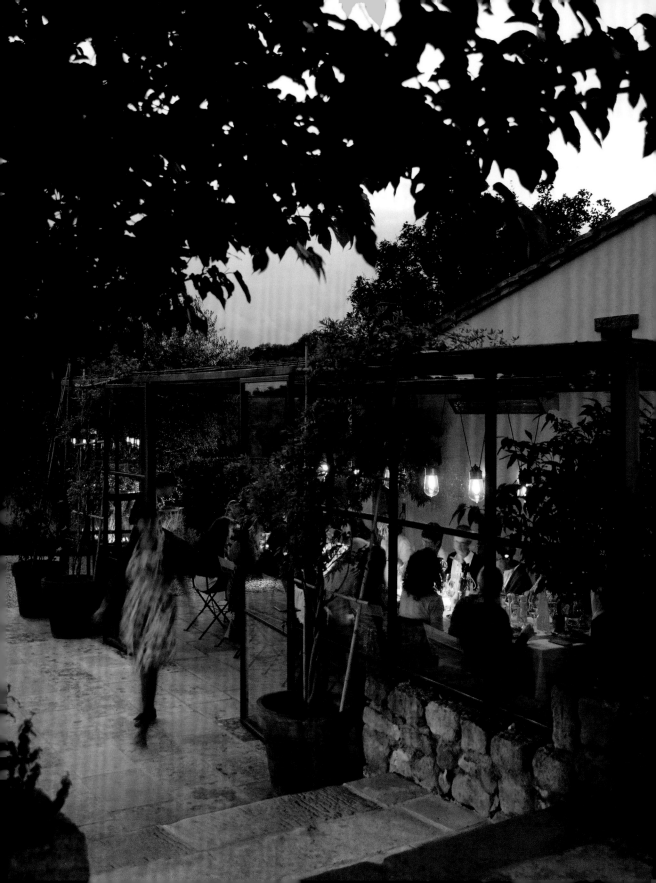

social media, and using various other apps. They spend an average of 30 percent of that time interacting on social media. I asked Sarah Urquhart, a coaching psychologist who specializes in the impact of device use on the brain, what all this time staring at our screens does to us. She told me something I already had an inkling of: the majority of time we spend on our devices is "spare time." Standing in line at the supermarket, sitting on the train heading to work, waiting for whatever, we scroll, text, play games and flip through messages. "Once upon a time, we were able to simply do nothing," Sarah said, "but we are now seeking constant stimulation and connection. In return, we seem to be losing the ability to just daydream, relax in our thoughts and open ourselves up to creative thinking."

We are social beings at heart. I know I'm stating the obvious when I say that social media feeds our craving to belong because it lets us connect with others with similar passions all around the world, as well as keep in touch with friends and family. But there are a lot of negatives attached too, one of which Sarah bluntly outlined: "It is like bonding ourselves to a robot, rather than with another human." The other big negative is that we can become obsessed, not only with comparing our own lives to others', but also with chasing likes and followers. If we have no one coming over on the weekend to hang out with us, but 25,000 followers on Twitter, are we really connected? I know what my Tuscan neighbours would say.

Sarah told me there is also an effect on the brain, called "cropping," among heavy device users. "This is brain shrinkage caused by the repetitive behaviour of constantly swiping and drifting through the Internet," she says. "If we are spending too much time surfing, we are not stimulated by normal everyday things." A walk in the woods over uneven ground, for instance, uses more of our brain and senses than watching the most stimulating YouTube video. She also explained that our willpower is adversely affected when we're exhausted by constant distraction: "For example, the advertisements running up and down on our digital screens pull us away from the task at hand. Our eyes, quite understandably, seek the excitement of something new. Watching a movie while flicking through Instagram and checking Facebook is not good for the brain. It drains us, which in turn affects our will to undertake other activities that matter. As a result, we make less favorable decisions about our diet, movement and real interaction."

Many of us—and especially women, in my experience—love to talk about their ability to multi-task, viewing it almost as a badge of honour. I, for one, consider myself a gold medallist at multi-tasking. But as it turns out, our brains do not function at an optimal level when doing a million things at once. Rather, they work best when focused on one task at a time. That's the antithesis of how you live when you are at the beck and call of devices.

Do You Really Need to Answer That Now?

Our digital world has made us more impatient, more impulsive. We think we need immediate answers. If we don't get an instant reply to an e-mail, we leap to conclusions: they don't like us, the deal has gone south, they're ignoring us—how rude! And it's usually completely untrue. We need to build behaviours that help us relearn patience, such as no phones on the dining table or by the bed. Find strategies that help you resist the temptation to drift mindlessly around the world on the Internet— or risk the brain shrinkage Sarah described.

Forge Face-to-Face Connections

Our devices connect us to the world, but we need to reassert our actual connections to the neighbourhood we live in and the people around us. Try moving the chat room to your living room. It sounds crazy, but this is how I made a life in Tuscany, where at first I knew not a soul. I used social media to find other expats who'd fallen in love with the Tuscan lifestyle like I had. It does take guts to say hello through Instagram and ask whether someone would like to meet you for a coffee. It's rather like going on a blind date. But everyone I reached out to has become someone I can call a friend. For that, I do thank my devices.

Take a Digital Vacation

I am not a fan of a full digital detox. I believe it's unrealistic to go cold turkey. I think I could give up wine more easily than my phone. Really. But we are capable of functioning without our devices for a period of time, and for the sake of our health and well-being, we should find ways and times to shut them down. Irony of ironies, you might find you need one of the many apps designed to track how much time you spend on your devices and remind you to take a break.

Baby steps are key. Try a no-device lunch break. Grab the usual sandwich, but instead of eating as you scroll on your phone, find a quiet bench and do nothing but taste the food and watch the world go by. If you're incapable of resisting temptation, try leaving your phone behind. It'll feel weird at first—like you're missing a limb— but if you do it, you will likely find that your device-free break has revived your energy for the afternoon ahead.

Once you've mastered the digital-free lunch hour, try for a whole weekend off the grid. If you like to bake, set aside the hours you need to make something, then share it with a neighbour. Dance, write, read a book—anything other than turning on a device. (You may have to tell your family this is what you are up to so they don't worry when you don't answer their texts.) See if you feel like our guests at the villa do: happy that you turned that darn thing off.

Don't let the Internet's many benefits and entertainments dim your own precious life. The time spent surfing can be fun and educational, but what could you be doing instead? Take back some of those hours and use them to get out into the real world and to spend more time fully engaged with those you love.

Bring Back the Notebook

Laptops and phones have invaded the workplace and the classroom, but if you're looking for a less distracted, more connected way to be in the world, set them aside when talking with people. In business meetings, jot down notes the old-fashioned way,

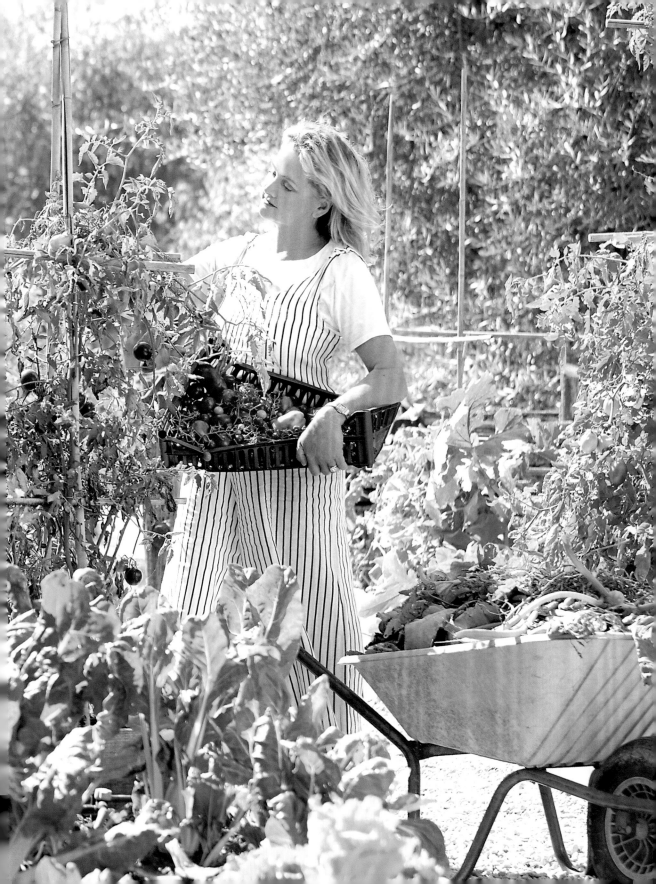

with pen and paper. Scribbling is so much more impressive than tapping, and writing something by hand reinforces what you're trying to remember way more effectively than typing on a keyboard. I love the story I heard about a school-teacher who reinforced a phone ban in his class with a sign on the blackboard that said he knew if the students were texting because humans do not otherwise stare at their laps.

Create a Healthy Digital Relationship

I work hard at this. I love Instagram—both sharing a little of my goings-on with strangers and seeing what others are getting up to. But I know myself well, so I set limits: ten minutes in the morning to post and thirty minutes in the evening to surf. That's it. By limiting myself, I enjoy it more. I also turn off the automatic notifications that trigger my "I want to know more" impulses.

When I'm out with friends, I put my phone away—out of sight, not on the table. If you are going out for dinner, go out for dinner. The world will not stop functioning if you spend two hours eating and catching up with your partner or friends. *But what about emergencies?* you ask. True emergencies are rare. *What if the kids call?* That's one I've heard myself say, but the little ones have a babysitter (who will know how to reach you in a crisis), and if the older ones are calling, nine times out of ten it's because they want to borrow some money or the car. *What about work?* Many workplaces, aware of digital overload and burnout, now have an after-hours policy of no business communications. If you have a work emergency or deadline, you won't be out for dinner in the first place. And otherwise, the office can wait.

I also suggest removing news apps from your devices. It is important to be informed, but the old saying "What we don't know won't hurt us" is so true. If the world is about to come to an end, someone will tell you. Being constantly tapped into the news raises our stress levels.

Be conscious of how cellphone time makes you feel. Is it useful and energizing, or does it leave you feeling drained and stressed? Do the feeds of particular "friends" leave you irritated or feeling worthless? Each of us needs to work out for ourselves which elements of the digital world are right for us and which undermine our energy and our joy in life. The latter are the ones we need to learn to avoid!

How to Bring Tuscany Home

- Make your digital world a healthy one.
- Try to turn some of your online friends into off-line ones.
- Try at least a partial digital detox. Start by noting your emotions after a marathon on your devices. Do you feel good to be alive, or drained of energy? Use your personal responses as a guide to what to keep and what to cut.
- Reduce online time and replace it with me time.
- Make a strict rule in your home that all phones are turned off during mealtimes, and support restaurants that try to do the same.
- Do not sleep with your phone beside the bed. As I advised in Lesson 3, put it in another room. Use an old-fashioned alarm clock instead of your phone's alarm.
- Either lose the news apps or make sure their notifications are switched off.

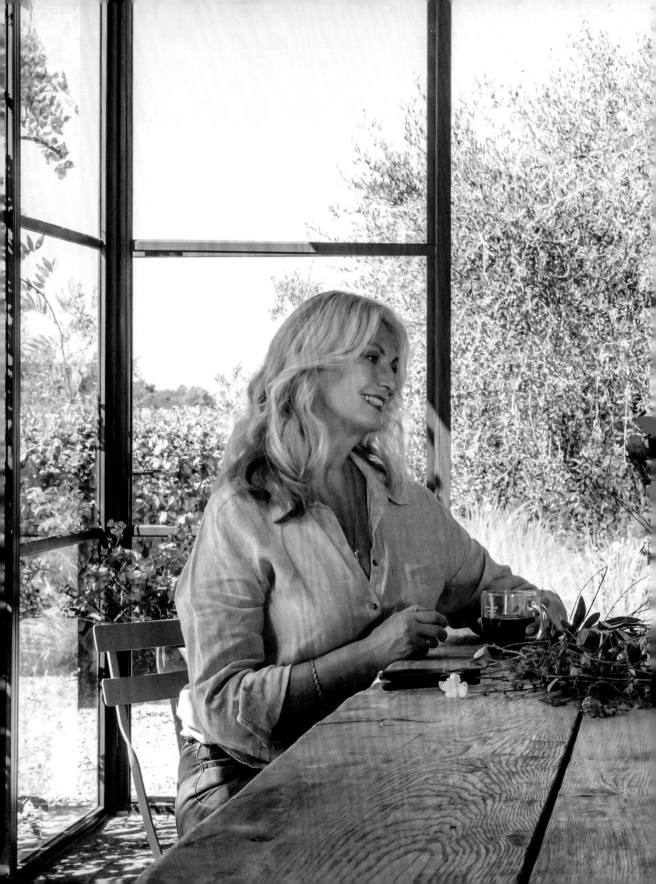

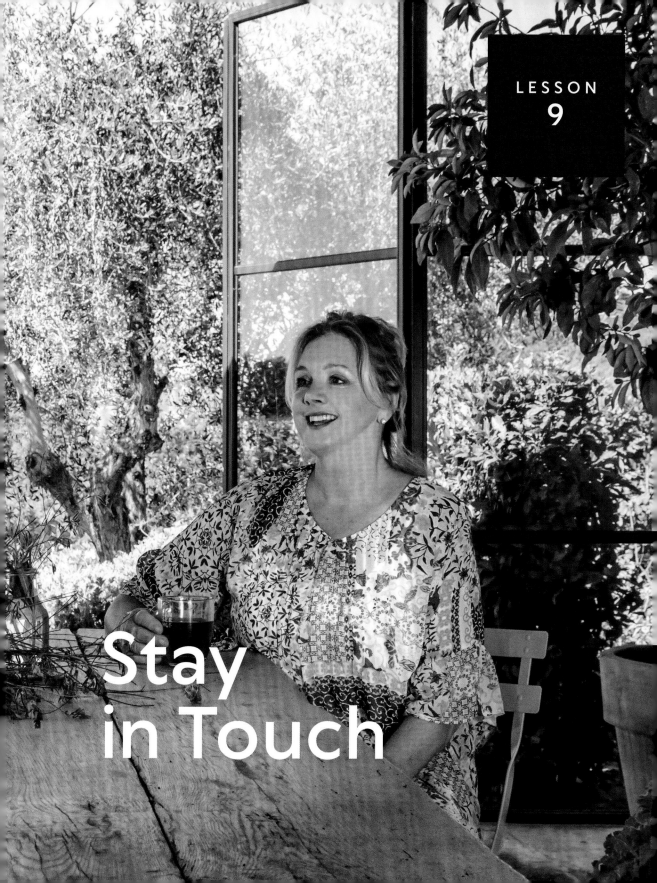

Stay in Touch

Italians Love to Hug

ABBRACCI E BACI—HUGS AND KISSES—WHAT WE ALL LONG FOR. Over the last year, it's been up in the air as to whether this vital custom will come back into our lives after the pandemic. Here in Italy, will I ever again be greeted with a kiss on both cheeks? I am sure they will return. We humans need to touch!

Any newcomer to Italy soon notices how comfortable people are in each other's company. They like to stand close to one another when talking, to plant a kiss on a cheek or reach out to lay a hand on an arm, and they often walk hand in hand. They already know something that billions of people around the world realized during the COVID-19 crisis: the importance of physical contact. When all of a sudden we couldn't give or receive a simple hug, or even a handshake, it was disorienting for everyone; for some, it had a real impact on their mental health. It makes sense, given that touch is our first sense, developing in the womb, and that friendships, relationships and trust are reinforced by our primal need to reach out to others.

To the Italians, touch is an essential part of how they communicate. This is especially clear on the weekly market days, which bring the entire town out onto the street. I love the food stalls piled with fruits and vegetables, the succulent olives glistening alongside slippery balls of burrata driven up from Naples that morning, aged pecorino cheeses piled to toppling heights alongside banks of local herbs. Numerous porchetta vans serving up savoury roast pork vie for business with tables laden with lacy underwear and others selling tractor parts. But it's the people-watching that captivates me. Old men kissing each other on wrinkled foreheads. Little girls skipping arm in arm. Teenagers constantly hugging, poking and roughhousing with each other. Women nose to nose in deep conversation, giving understanding pats on the back. Arms are stroked, hands held and hair gently smoothed back off a friend's forehead.

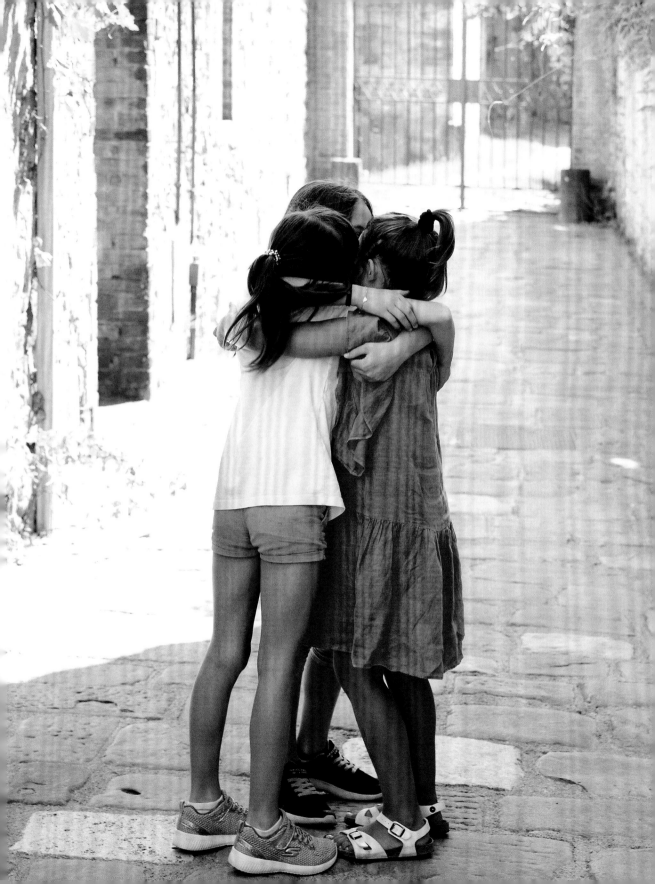

At first, all this casual touching unsettled me because it was so different from the English reserve I was used to. But I also found it profoundly moving and intriguing, and now it seems as natural as breathing—at least when I'm in Italy. Comfort levels with human touch are as diverse in different cultures as are their cuisines. We all know what it feels like when touch is given and received awkwardly, inappropriately and wrongly. That happens even in Italy: just ask any young tourist who has ever had an Italian man follow her down a street in Rome, looking for an opportunity to pinch her backside. Yet overall, the Italians have much to teach us about the way touch, freely given and received, offers healing and comfort and strengthens the bonds of friendship.

Still, what's normal and well-meant in Italy can be quite a shock to someone new to the country. For instance, when my colleague Penny came over from New York to talk about a new project, she'd never been to Italy before. Although she must have been tired from the flight and the time change, she got to the villa on a quintessential warm Tuscan evening, and she was keen to see the surrounding area. We wandered up to the local village just as our numerous neighbours were out for their *passeggiata*. As is the custom, I waved to everyone we passed. When I saw Fabio, a kind man who is one of the pillars of the community, leaning against the wall of his old stone cottage, I decided to introduce him to Penny. Fabio stepped forward and gave her a big squeeze on both arms, then an enthusiastic hug, followed by a kiss on both cheeks. Penny froze, completely horrified! I quickly rescued her from Fabio's well-intended greeting and, waving goodbye to him, rushed her to the safer ground of the bar. As she calmed down over a drink, she explained how incredibly alien she found it for a complete stranger to be so physically familiar.

Fast-forward five days. After a busy week brainstorming together, inspired by the beauty of the landscape, I took Penny to the airport for her flight home. As she was leaving, she told me how moved she'd been by the tactile warmth of the Tuscans. "It just seems so natural now," she said. "And I am going to hug more—hug like an Italian!"

Countless studies show the importance of touch to our health and well-being. Still, there are those who simply don't like being touched. Over the last decade, with growing consciousness of childhood sexual abuse and the widespread sexual power dynamics sharply highlighted by the #MeToo Movement, many walls have been raised against touching each other. Most women I know have stories of the creepy guy at the office or the over-familiar "friend" whose uninvited physical attentions were inappropriate or worse. So there are good reasons why, at our workplaces and schools, we should think twice before touching each other in support and love, and make sure to ask permission.

The downside is that recent research tells us people are now suffering because so much casual touch is off limits. This was explained eloquently by Dr. Jon Reeves, a clinical psychologist from Seattle, who said, "Touch is our first language and one of our core needs. The touch of a safe, trusted loved one can alleviate anxiety and promote a sense of well-being all on its own."

At times, everyone needs a gentle pat on the shoulder or a full-on reassuring hug; it is a biological fundamental. Thankfully, a growing number of teenagers in North America are bucking the no-touch policy. They greet each other with a hug, just as my Italian friends do: guys hugging guys, girls hugging girls, everyone saying hello by wrapping their arms around each other. They've even named their hugs. There is the wrap-your-arms-around-someone, typical "friend hug," the "thump hug," which begins with a bang on the back and moves into a fist bump, and even a "bear claw hug," where your elbows jut out, apparently. Oh, those teenagers!

Psychologists and businesses have been stepping into the void, turning our need for touch into an industry, with cuddle clinics popping up alongside hug therapists. In Japan, there are cuddle cafés where, for a fee, you can receive a long embrace from an expert hugger. I know—the world seems to have gone mad! But for some people, it can be excruciatingly painful to reach out physically, so maybe there is a need for professional huggers.

I am heartened that more of us non-Italians, including medical researchers, now acknowledge the importance of touch. That certainly wasn't the case when I was a girl. My best friend, Rosie, and I were inseparable in school and on weekends. We just loved being together, whether we were snuggled under a blanket doing homework or brushing each other's hair. We sat together in class and often stroked each other's palm with a wooden ruler, which we found weirdly comforting, especially during our grade four geography class as the teacher, boring Mr. Skinner, droned on and on. One day we were caught in the act. The teacher confiscated the ruler and sent us to the headmistress's office, where she disciplined us for indulging in this innocent pleasure with whacks from the same ruler. She hurt us, and worse, she made us ashamed of something that was completely innocent. A child in that position today would not receive corporal punishment, but touch amongst youngsters is still frowned on in schools. Yes, children need to learn when touch is inappropriate—and from whom—but they shouldn't lose out on the wonders of an impulsive embrace as a way to communicate comfort, reassurance and affection. The lack of such touch stresses us all out, and especially children, I would argue, who are still figuring out how to navigate the world.

The Healing Power of Touch

Here at the villa, the food, vistas and fresh air are major factors in raising our guests' levels of joy, but as the week goes on, the healing power of touch also comes into play. I keep a photograph on my desk of two of the women on one of our first Tuscan getaways, casually strolling hand in hand down a wooded path through dappled sunlight, all barriers between them vanished. The picture fills me with sweet emotion because I know these two were strangers only three days earlier!

LALLA

Lalla is special to us here, not just because she is a kindly soul, but because of the pleasure, peace and joy she gives everyone who is lucky enough to be massaged by her strong hands. Lalla, an Italian, fell in love with Ayurveda—an ancient Indian medical practice that fosters the balance of mind, body and spirit—while travelling through Kerala, in the south of India, years ago. The region is known as the home of Ayurveda, so while she was there, Lalla treated herself to a massage using these ancient techniques. She had her "aha!" moment about what she would do with her life while lying face down on the traditional wooden therapy table as two female practitioners simultaneously poured warm scented oil over her naked body and set to work with all four hands in a rhythmic massage that she found weird and exotic at first.

As she began to relax and enjoy the experience, she became aware of a startling difference between the touch of the two women. One of them seemed fully engaged, her hands at one with Lalla's body and being. The other seemed like she was just going through the motions. The touch of the fully engaged therapist reminded Lalla of her mother's warmth and intimacy, and how she and her mother connected through touch. After her massage was over, she approached this therapist and asked to be taught the technique. She trained for months with her massage therapist, and then set off across India to meet and learn from other Ayurvedic gurus.

Now we all benefit from Lalla's unique massages, which blend the passion of the Italian people with ancient Indian Ayurveda. All in a hut on a Tuscan hillside.

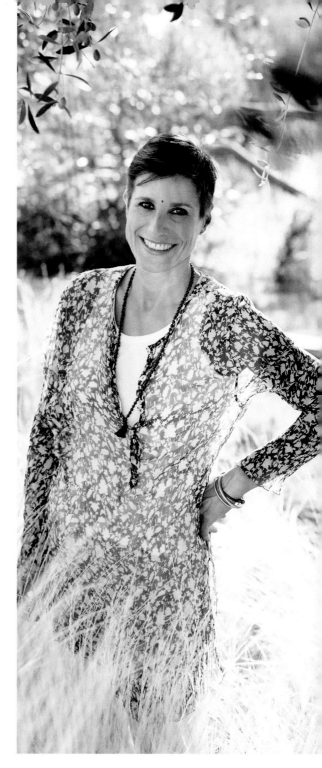

As friendships form here, you can measure the growing trust and confidence between the women by the number of hugs they give, the arm they drape around another's shoulders and the spontaneous kisses of greeting.

We supplement this particular type of touch medicine with the treatments our massage therapist, Lalla, offers to each guest, designed to release stress and toxicity from the body. Lalla's rhythmic technique, which involves applying various levels of pressure and copious amounts of warm oils, can be quite the surprise to a woman who ventures into her hut for the first time, vulnerably naked under a bathrobe except for a pair of flimsy paper knickers. And I have seen a plethora of reactions: floods of tears as Lalla's touch releases deep-rooted emotions, bashful giggles from women whose limbs are now as relaxed as jelly, quiet smiles as if some special secret has been shared. Lalla specializes in Ayurvedic massage, not the deep-tissue massage that is more common in Europe and North America. Rather than digging into the muscles, she stimulates the entire surface of the skin with hands in constant motion. Her massages feel like receiving a long, heartwarming embrace.

What we eat nourishes the body, and so does touch. It may not be as critical to our immediate survival, but it's just as important to our well-being, benefiting both the person on the receiving end and the one offering it. Contact with another living creature, from a horse to a hamster—it doesn't even have to be a person!—brings us comfort and lowers our stress levels, which is why care homes bring dogs (and even ponies) in to visit the residents. Emotional support dogs go a step beyond the usefulness of guide dogs and have become an important means of caring for people recovering from trauma, both physical and mental, and children with learning disorders, among others.

Deep inside, no matter our age, we are all still that toddler who needs a cuddle to help make the world feel safe. So try to remember what the Italians never forget, and reach out and touch someone.

How to Bring Tuscany Home

- Start a touch journal. Make a note of the number of times each day you give a welcomed hug to someone. Add them up at the end of the week. Can you reach out even more?

- Don't forget the elderly. It's easy to show affection to a child, but our elders are greatly in need of tenderness as well.

- Follow in the Italians' footsteps and use touch as a form of communication and reassurance. This may strike certain people as inappropriate, so ask permission and explain why you'd like to reach out to them. They may say yes, and you will both feel better.

- Add a hug or a pat on the back to any praise you give. It will mean so much more.

- Always honour each other's personal space. Due to a past experience or a cultural difference, some of us really do not like to be touched.

- Experiment with different types of massages until you find one that works for you. Massage is beneficial not just to our achy muscles but also for our entire physical and mental well-being.

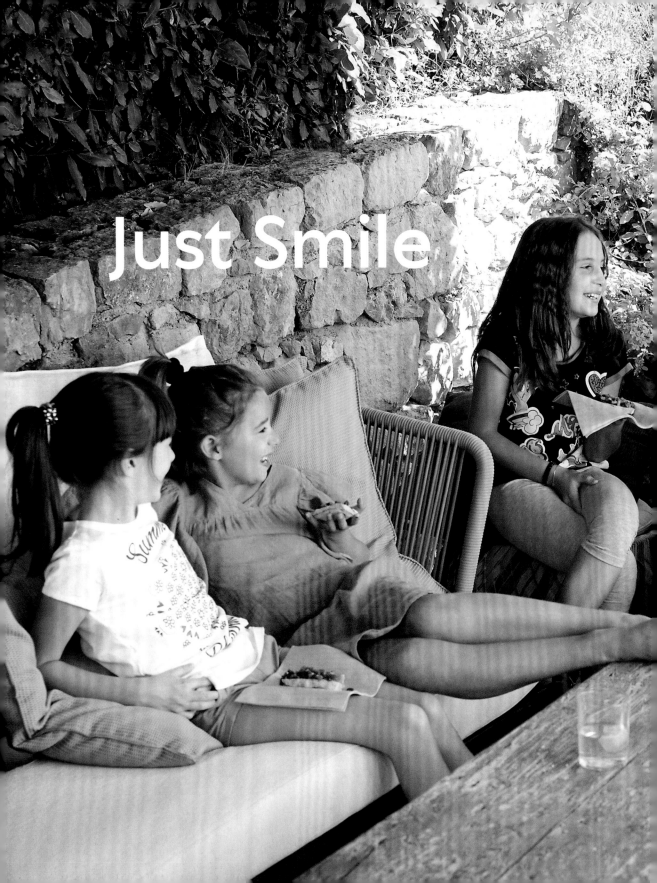

Just Smile

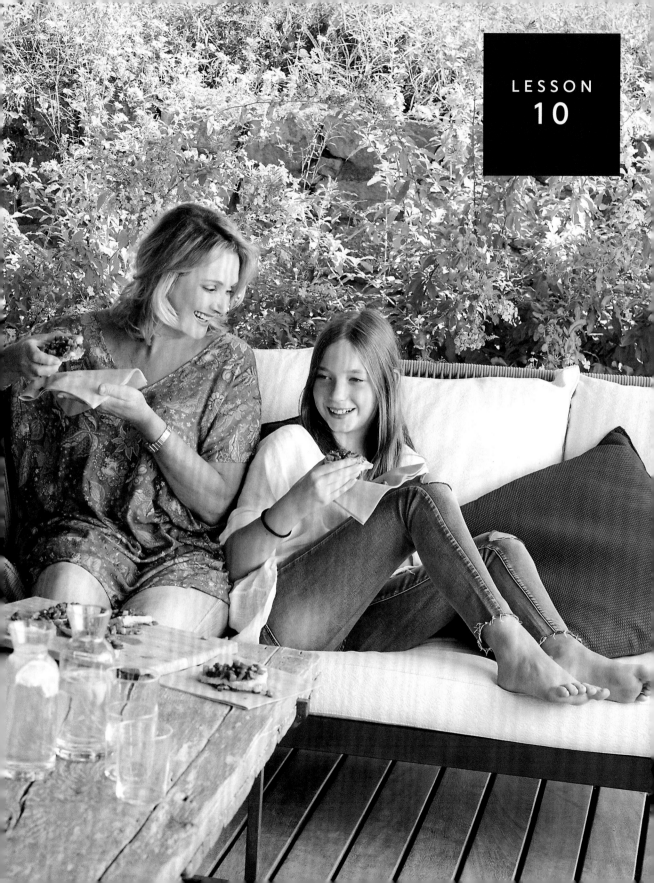

The Happy House

FINALLY, DEAR FRIENDS, I OFFER THE SIMPLEST LESSON OF ALL: just smile, as many times a day as you can. That grinning emoji you tack to the end of texts is all very well, but try shifting it off your device and onto your beautiful face. There is so much value in a smile. It enriches us beyond measure, yet costs nothing to give. It is our simplest gift to the world—our joy. A smile expresses happiness and satisfaction and fosters goodwill.

Louis Armstrong sang the brilliant line, "When you smile, the world smiles with you." Smiling *is* contagious. It's hard not to smile back at someone who smiles at you. Smiles are a silent language that can communicate a multitude of things, all of them good. Hearts melt when a newborn smiles for the first time. A smile offers forgiveness, no words needed. A smile dulls fear and can soften pain. Sometimes all it takes to regain your joy in life is the gift of a smile.

I smile a lot. Even if deep inside I don't feel quite as exuberant as my grin suggests, I keep working those facial muscles because I find that smiling actually improves my mood. Smiling is a habit. If you're not a natural smiler, work at it; slowly but surely, you'll notice a shift in the way the world opens to you.

One of our guests at the villa, Georgia, was widowed way too young, about six months before she came to Tuscany. Her husband had been planning to join her on the retreat, but was killed in a car crash. After some persuasion from her family, she decided to come on the trip alone. I was impressed with her grit, but I have to admit I was mystified about why she looked so happy after such a heartbreaking experience. Georgia's answer will stay with me forever. "I could not bear to see the pitiful reflection of myself in the eyes of all those concerned," she said. "It had to stop. So I began to dig very deep inside myself to summon a smile when I talked to others. In time, I had to dig a little less, and finally it became normal to hold on to a brighter disposition. The pain of losing him is relentless, but now I save the moments of

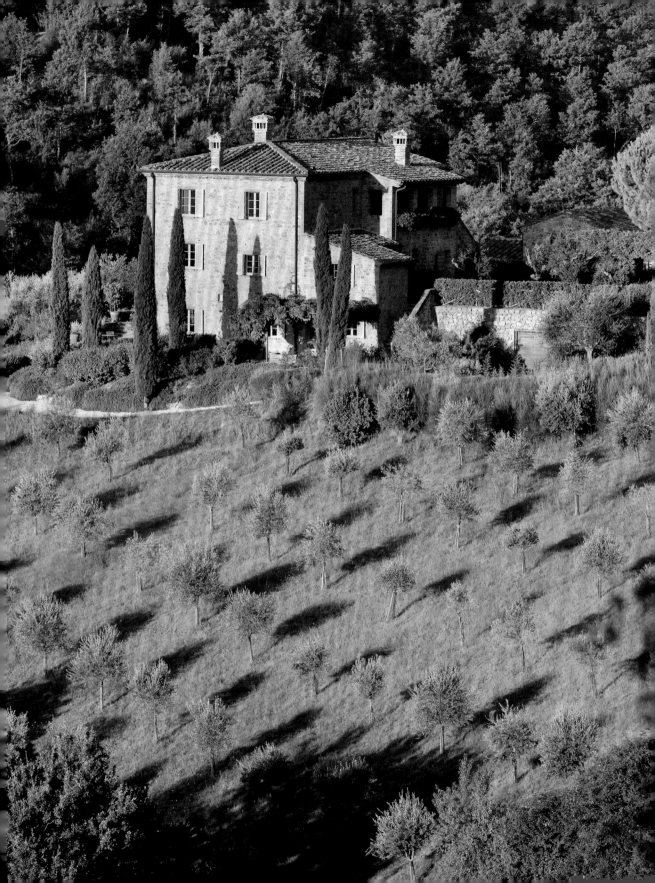

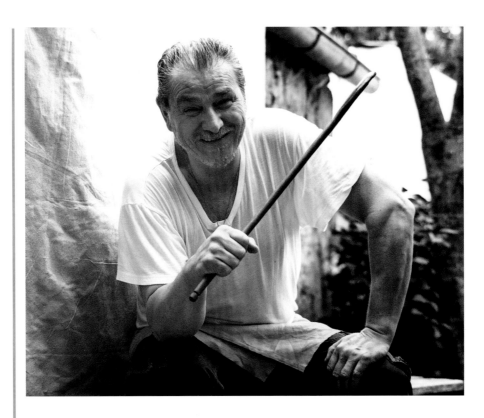

ALBO

Gobbi 13 (named after the hunchback who apparently guarded the village in the thirteenth century) appears to be an unassuming eatery, but don't be fooled—it is a landmark in the area. Dining there last week, my eyes followed Albo, *il proprietario*, smiling throughout the lunchtime crush. He clearly adored the regulars who were tucking into bowls of the day's special, and the old-timers beamed back at him. He treated the tourists with a similar smiling appreciation for their taste in choosing his joint. He takes immense pleasure in feeding the room, and in return the eaters pay homage to him by packing the place every day. The restaurant is a family affair, and the food is classic trattoria, simple and scrumptious.

As we paid the bill, which seemed meagre for such a feast, I told him, "You never, ever stop smiling!" Planting a kiss on my cheek, he grinned even more. He said, "My uncomplaining wife does all the cooking, my son serves the food, so what purpose do I have but to smile—that is my job."

I asked him, then, if it was an act to keep the customers happy. "*Assolutamente no!*" he cried. "I don't feel fully dressed without my smile. It is my gift to the hungry customers."

intense sadness for when I allow myself to fall apart, and then, believe me, I let go."
She was living proof of how tenacious one has to be when working on happiness.

Around here, our villa's nickname is "*la casa felice*," or "the happy house." One day, while drinking my morning cappuccino, I decided to ask Tomas, the barista, how the locals came to call it that. Tomas pointed over my shoulder. When I turned to look, there was Jacky's husband, Steve Brown (a world-renowned record producer), leading a gaggle of our guests on an early-morning trek as the women babbled and giggled like animated children. "Everyone who comes in here from your villa is always smiling, always happy," Tomas said. I take that as the ultimate compliment. Our whole aim is to send people home with the new tools for a life of renewed vitality—one of them being to smile more.

Make It a Habit

How many times has someone asked you if you're okay when you're actually just fine? You might be feeling at one with the universe, but your face is telling a different story, appearing stern, sad or disengaged. This impression can get worse with aging as the facial muscles move south. All the surgery in the world won't bring back our youthful freshness, but a smile lifts everything—it's the least-expensive beauty remedy of all.

JACKY SAYS

Dopamine, serotonin and endorphins are all released when you smile, and they all reduce your levels of cortisol. Your body relaxes, and your heart rate and blood pressure are lowered. When someone smiles at you, you tend to automatically smile back, a reflex controlled by a section of the brain called the cingulate cortex, part of the autonomic nervous system and the limbic system, which regulates our emotions. Studies have shown that the sight of a smiling face activates the orbitofrontal cortex, the region in the brain that processes sensory rewards. So when you see a person smiling at you, you feel rewarded and smile back. Other studies have found that practising smiling can help train the brain to have a more positive outlook.

Begin by asking yourself how many times a day you smile. If you have no clue, ask a friend or colleague how they would rank you on the smile index. If they say not so high, especially when you think you smile a lot, you have your work cut out for you.

Scientists have studied the physical and emotional aspects of smiling and how our facial expressions affect us and those around us. Think of a teacher who looks miserable. Will they be able to hold the attention of the class as successfully as a teacher who punctuates their lectures with smiles? A sullen server in a first-class restaurant can ruin the meal no matter how delicious the food. A flight attendant sharing the warmth of a smile makes the flight seem less onerous, even if we're stuck in the back row of the plane, next to the loo. Smiling is a sign of respect and attentiveness you show to others, and with practice it can easily become a habit. While it may seem phony at first to "work" on your smile, if you keep on trying, gradually your practice smiles will turn real, and actual happiness will blossom.

I'm fascinated by the way different cultures use smiles as a form of greeting. On my first trip to India, I was mesmerized by people offering a sideways nod of hello, accompanied by the widest of smiles. People in Thailand bow to you, hands together, and offer a gentle smile. Italians keep me grinning because they love to smile. Though not always. If a Tuscan villager doesn't recognize you, they will stare and frown, which I've learned to translate as *Hmm, who is this person in my neigh-bourhood, what do they want, where are they going and who are they visiting?* But if you counteract that stare with a sunny smile, their dark thoughts seem to immediately evaporate and they beam back at you from ear to ear.

When I settled into life on my Tuscan hillside, I was defeated in my smiling counter-offensive by only one neighbour, an ancient woman known as Frangolina (a nickname meaning "strawberry"), whom I would often encounter dragging her thick-stockinged legs up the hill as she carried an armful of sticks. Try as I might, she never smiled back. Eventually, I realized she was nicking the sticks, gathered from my little forest, from the villa's woodpile. The nerve of her!

Returning from a walk one day, I saw her shuffling towards me. When she spotted me, she stopped, laid down the bunch of sticks and draped her threadbare cardigan over them as if that would somehow hide them, then looked up at me with feigned innocence. I offered her my brightest smile. She paused for what seemed an age, then returned a wide, toothless grin. I gathered up her bundle and walked alongside her to a tiny cottage. Ducking through a low doorway into her hobbit-like home, she took the bundle from me, then flung some of the newly stolen wood onto the open fire. Motioning for me to sit, she handed me a sticky glass of homemade Vin Santo. It was overly syrupy and a little gritty, but I politely sipped away as she reminisced about growing up in this house, and about the forest I viewed as "mine." She had once crouched there in the bracken for days, hiding from German soldiers during the Second World War. She told me lighter stories, too, chortling wickedly about an old romance and even getting up to show me a dress she'd worn to someone's wedding eons ago. I only understood snippets, but I was riveted anyway because her smiling, wrinkled face was so beautiful. Two days later, I found a box of fresh eggs and a bunch of wildflowers on my doorstep. Looking up the road, I saw her carrying another batch of "my" wood back home.

We don't speak the same language, and we're from different generations and cultures, yet whenever we greet each other now, her wicked smile is worth a thousand words.

How to Bring Tuscany Home

- Practise smiling.
- Consciously increase the number of times you smile in a day.
- Carry a couple of images in your head that are guaranteed to make you smile, and resort to them when the need arises.
- Smile at a stranger for no reason. Chances are they'll smile back.
- Smile at a friend just because you like them.
- Try smiling when you're talking on the phone, even though there's no one there to see you. How does it affect you?
- Try to smile at your flaws and mistakes.
- Find at least one activity a day that has you beaming.

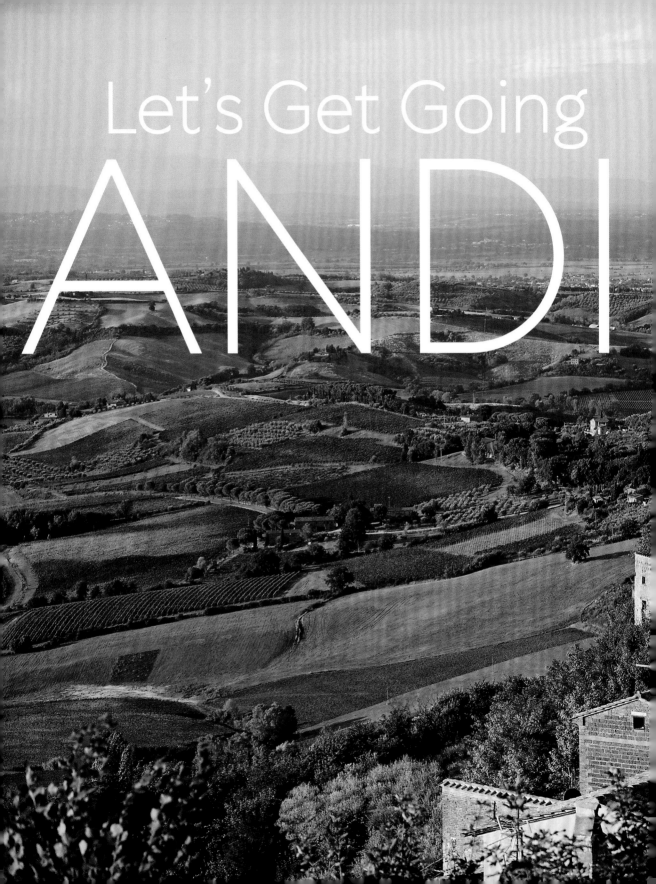

Let's Get Going
ANDI

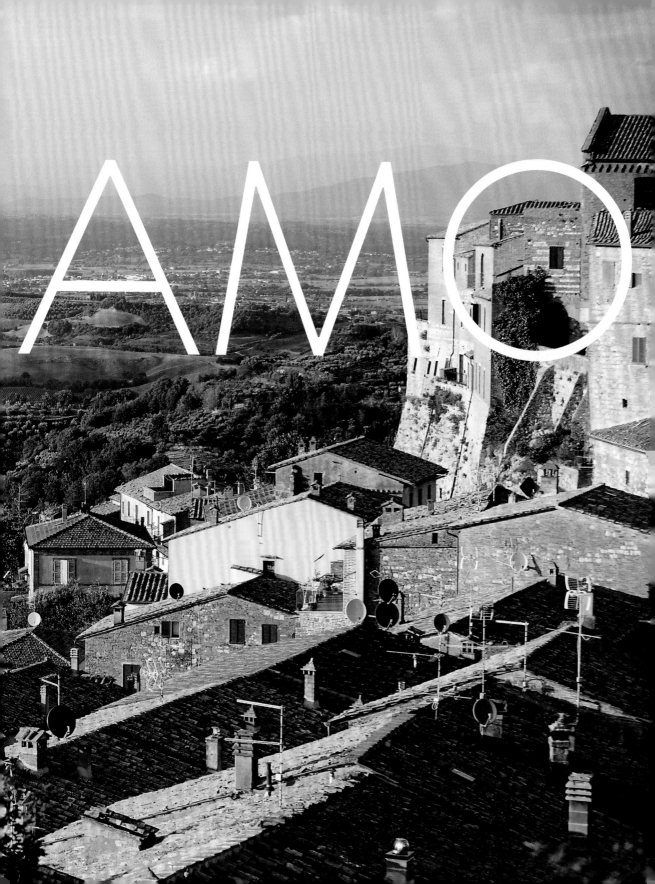

All the Ways We Can Truly Bring Tuscany Home

MANGIA BENE, RIDI SPESSO, AMA MOLTO—eat well, laugh often, love more. These are words I've tried to live by since I moved to Tuscany, and all the lessons I've shared in this book have been aimed at helping you incorporate them into your own life.

So there you are, with your hand-picked fruit bubbling on the stove, your countertops full of sterilized jamming jars, inviting a neighbour over for a bonding conversation to help build your community. Your devices are gathering dust. After you've returned home again and bottled the jam, you're planning an afternoon power nap so you'll be energized to greet new friends when they pop in for an *aperitivo*. At the gathering, you'll recruit people for tomorrow morning's foraging excursion and an afternoon of weeding the new communal vegetable garden on the condo roof. Before you fall asleep tonight, you'll slow down with an hour-long meditation, yoga and breathing session, which will lead to the sweetest of dreams.

Okay, stop! Let's remember the true Tuscan mantra: *piano, piano*. Slowly, slowly, people!

Change is hard, and if changes are going to stick, they have to be realistic. It may not be the right time to work on a solid eight hours of sleep, for instance, if you have a newborn baby in the house. And if you live in the inner city, foraging and nature walks could be hard to come by. So start your journey to more vitality and joy by acting first on the lessons that really resonate with you. Put aside the rest for later.

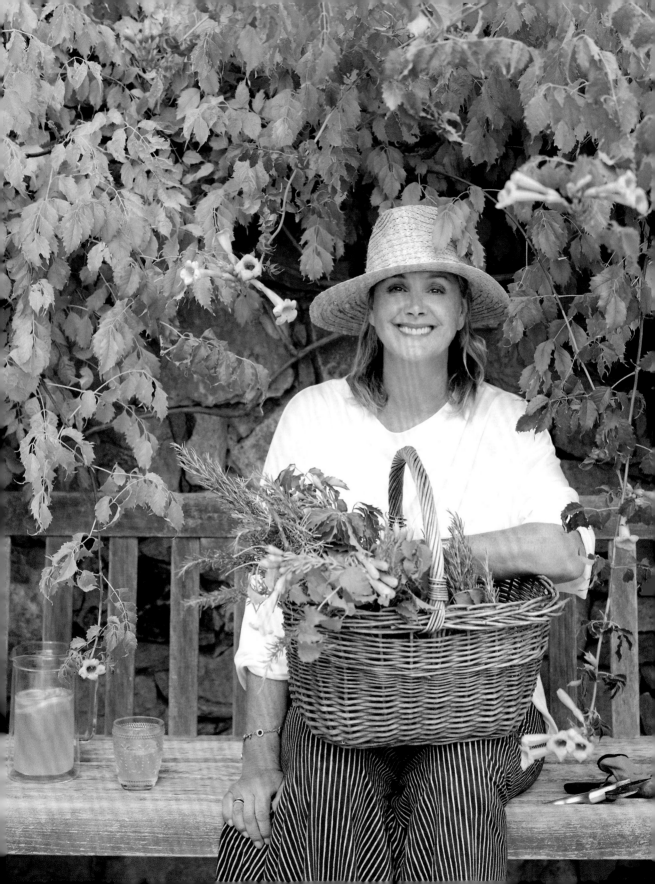

How to Break and Replace Habits

How do we make room in our lives to try a different way of living? We are creatures of habit, and our habits, both good and bad, affect us in every possible way, from the strength of our relationships to how well we age and how happy we feel. Understanding what triggers each habit is the key to changing it. Can you eat one potato chip? Not me. Knowing I'll be tempted, I simply don't buy them. I stock the fridge with containers of nibbles that do not spike my taste buds into endless munching. Become a detective who studies what drives your habits. The better you understand when and how harmful habits emerge and are reinforced, the better equipped you will be to defeat them.

What triggers a habit? A few years ago, at a party in England, I met a "habit" guru who helped people break bad habits. He said habits that are detrimental to our well-being often begin when we are bored or anxious. An excruciatingly long car trip on a highway, where you drive with only the company of other cars and the groomed landscape to look at, can have you eating masses of junk food to relieve the boredom. If you're worn out by a stressful job, you may feel like you have no energy on the weekend, so you numb yourself in front of the TV. The triggers are different for each of us.

Bad habits are tough to break, taking as much practice and repetition to undo as they did to form. Psychologists who specialize in this field work on four factors: the signal, the desire, the reaction and, finally, the reward. Imagine this scenario, drawn from my own loop of habits. Drained after a hectic day (the *signal* that I need to change my mood), I go to the fridge, where I find an open bottle of cold, crisp white wine. That's exactly what I *desire*, I think, and I reach for it, blocking any thoughts of easing my thirst with water—a better option. Before I can stop myself, I pour—the *reaction* to that initial signal. Sip, sip, and as the alcohol hits my stomach and passes into my bloodstream, I relax. That is my *reward* for working hard, or so I tell myself. The reward is important: it gratifies us, reinforcing the habit, bad or not.

If we know a habit is bad for us, we must try to break it, and to do this we need to disarm the trigger, redirect the craving and understand the reward. Work on one habit at a time. Plan ahead, to anticipate the craving. A square of dark chocolate after a meal is gratifying and possibly even good for us. Gobbling the whole bar? Not so good. Head that temptation off at the pass by having the small piece ready and waiting while tucking the rest away for another day. Out of sight, out of mind.

If you plan ahead and remove the initial trigger, chances are you'll be better able to control the craving, reducing its power over you. Don't leave that chilled screw-top bottle of wine in the fridge when you know it will call to you to open it. Replace it with a cold jug of gingered soda water. By removing the temptation ahead of time, you break the cycle and short-circuit the reward. It does not mean you will never enjoy a glass of white wine, only that you will become more conscious of why and how you're drinking it.

Let's say your triggers tell you that you can't get through the afternoon without the reward of a chocolate chip cookie—so tasty, but gradually adding inches around your middle. What you're really craving is not the cookie, but a break in the day's routine. Find something else to fill the gap. For a week, and then another week, and then a month, try to replace it with something even more soul-nourishing—a phone call to a favourite friend, perhaps. One month is not a huge amount of time in the scheme of things, and it will give you a chance to form a different habit, with better benefits.

A Doable Plan

Jacky tells me science has recognized that journaling—keeping a record of your diet, sleep patterns, habits and goals—is an extremely effective tool. Add five minutes to your bedtime routine and jot down the patterns of your day. This will help you recognize and eventually understand your triggers and your emotional states.

Everyone needs to find their own path to change, but Jacky and I thought we should end the book with a plan you can adopt and adapt to take our Tuscan lessons home. Remember, the Italian way is *slowly, slowly*, but steadily. With a bit of work, you'll be able to break your bad habits and replace them with ones that make you healthy, happy and full of joy.

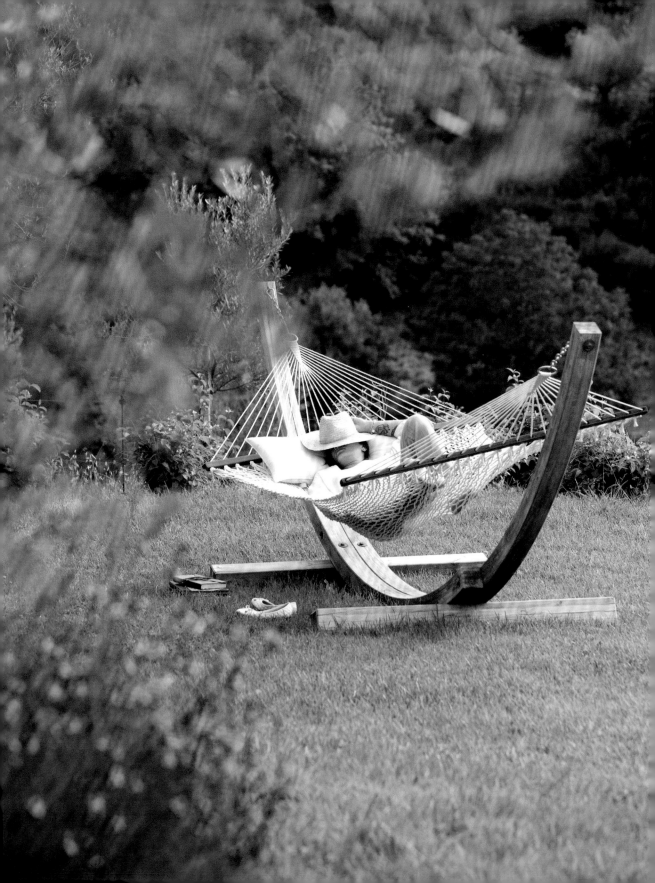

Month One

- Three times a week, find time for five or ten minutes of breathing exercises, mediation or yoga. This gives you a chance to just be, to do nothing—me time.
- Include vegetables with every meal. Have them ready to go in the fridge. Get into the habit of organizing healthy food options for the week ahead, and the temptation to grab the unhealthy stuff will melt away.
- Have at least one home-cooked meal a day. This can be prepared ahead of time and frozen, ready to warm up when needed.
- Walk for at least thirty minutes a day. Start with a spontaneous walk around the block at lunchtime, alone or with a colleague; before you know it, it will become a habit. Whether you're going solo or with company, walking calms the mind. It is a gift for our muscles and keeps joints supple by stimulating blood flow. Those knees and hips will thank you in later years.
- Once this month, reach out to someone from your past: a school friend, an old workmate, a relative. It can seem a little scary, I know, but the results may surprise you. Over the past ten years, I have tracked down many old buddies, even some from as far back as kindergarten. It is one of my proudest accomplishments, inviting old friends back into my life and being welcomed back into theirs. You won't regret it. Many such attempts will fizzle, but if just one old friendship is renewed, you both win.

Month Two

- Create a bedtime sleep routine and stick with it for a solid month. If after four weeks you're not sleeping any better, review Lesson 3 and keep trying. It does take time to change unhealthy sleep habits.

- Now let's get tougher: cut down the hours you spend on devices. Instead of scrolling, read a book while travelling to work. Leave your phone behind and get out on a bench at lunchtime, by yourself or with a friend, to watch the world go by. Stop fiddling around on the phone before bed. Leave it in another room. You'll soon feel the difference to your well-being and your sleep.

Month Three

By this time all these small changes should definitely have put a zip in your step. The challenge now is to add a few more:

- Begin this month by making a list of those around you who affect you in negative ways. Reduce the time you spend with them, even if you feel a deep obligation to them, familial or otherwise. There's no need to be cruel, of course. When you gain your equilibrium and can keep their impact on you in perspective, you may be able to spend more time together.
- Inventory your kitchen cupboards and throw out as much prepackaged food as you can bear to get rid of. In the villa, we have only one thin, tall, narrow cupboard of canned and dried goods to supply the entire mob of people who stay here. Peek inside and you will find dried beans, cans of tuna (for emergencies), coffee and teas, and about twenty cans of Canadian maple syrup that we offer as gifts to the locals (they love it). We also have a cool area in which we keep bottled homemade sauces and jams, which leads to my next suggestion . . .
- Choose a month when your local fruits and vegetables are abundant and host a preserving and sauce-making party. Pour your heart and soul into it, and even make it an annual event. It's a beautiful way to bond with your friends and make new ones—and to create ready-to-go food for the year ahead.
- Swap big supermarket shopping trips for food services that deliver fresh local produce. They can be more expensive, for sure, but you'll waste less and avoid the temptation of impulse buys, so you'll find that you actually save some money in these ways.

Month Four, and Forever

Our passions and purpose ebb and flow through the years. But if you've realized that you're constantly living on the lower rungs of that old olive-picking ladder (see page 49), it's time to push yourself to find new passions and new purpose. Work hard at this renewal of self—dig deep, educate yourself, meet people, be curious. Do not be afraid to make changes. The way forward is there, waiting for you.

The most important lesson of all? Make a robust effort to grow a tribe. Join everything; get to know your neighbours. Study those around you who have glowing skin, a healthy outlook and a smile for all. Yes, they likely eat well and exercise often, but I'd wager the source of their joy is engagement with their community. Modern living can strip away our connections, leaving us alone in our own bubble. We must embrace authenticity, physical touch and eye-to-eye contact.

So strategize, plan and take your time incorporating our ten Tuscan lessons into a daily routine. Tick off every achievement, and glory in it. You will have earned it, and it won't be just you who benefits, but everyone you know.

As I write this, my sweet Hans has run up to the village to pick up pesto from the *alimentari* for a pasta lunch. Eleonora makes her pesto fresh on Wednesdays, and Hans tells me hers is better than mine. He has been gone for two hours now, and I know why. He is lingering at the counter with the *nonnas*, gossiping—probably about the same thing they talked about yesterday. He is making sure they are all served before he is, because he is in his happy place, communing with our neighbours. He'll eventually come home, with or without the pesto, but surely with a story or two.

This is the heart of the joy we've found here. And it is a feeling you can create anywhere if you take the time, have the desire and study the Tuscan way.

ANGELINA

Bisnonna Angelina is ninety-four years young and beautiful, with a twinkle in her eye and a carefree mind. She landed in London in 1947 as a newlywed. She'd met her Scottish soldier husband during the war, and with Europe devastated and her hometown of Rome in tatters, she settled down in our big-city London neighbourhood. She lives across the street from me, in a small Georgian row house like mine, and Jacky lives one street over. The three of us have many a doorstep chat, and Jacky and I always learn something from her.

As a young woman, far from home, Angelina recreated the *dolce vita* in London. She is the epitome of the Italian generosity of spirit and everything else this book is about. Everyone around here knows her name. She has befriended the Turkish barber, the Indian baker, the Jamaicans who run the café and the little ones at the nursery school on the corner. She regularly hops on the bus to visit the local shops, buying supplies for the Italian feasts she still cooks for anyone who will join her. She has created her own familiar community within an English city very different from the one where she grew up. She is curious about everything and lives with purpose. She smiles a great deal, and people smile back at her.

What a pleasure it is to spend time with Angelina, who is so full of passion and kindness. She successfully transplanted her rich Italian ways to another country—showing us that if we are part of a community, if we eat well and sleep soundly, and most of all if we feel that we have purpose, we too can live long lives filled with joy.

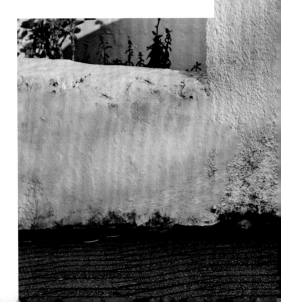

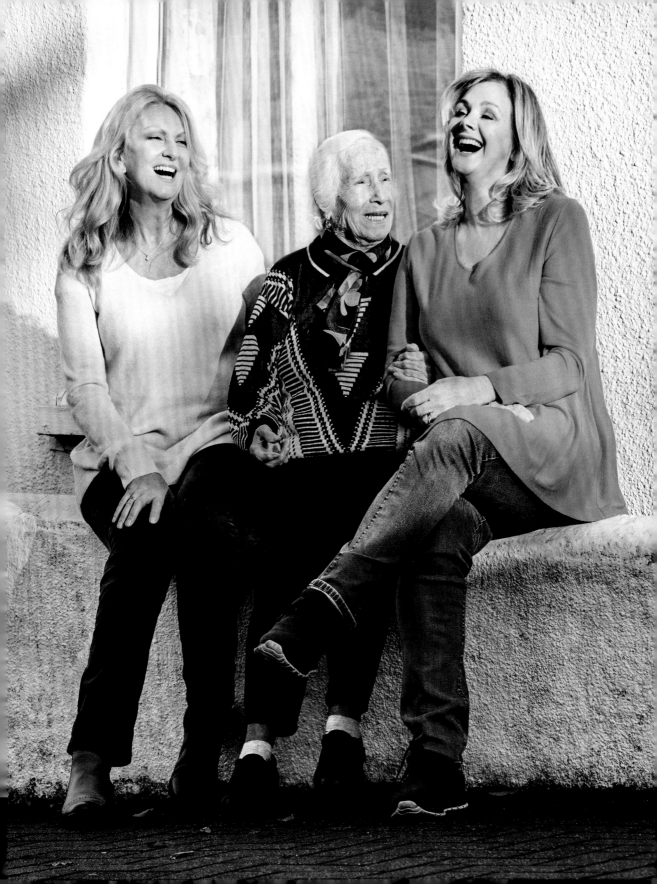

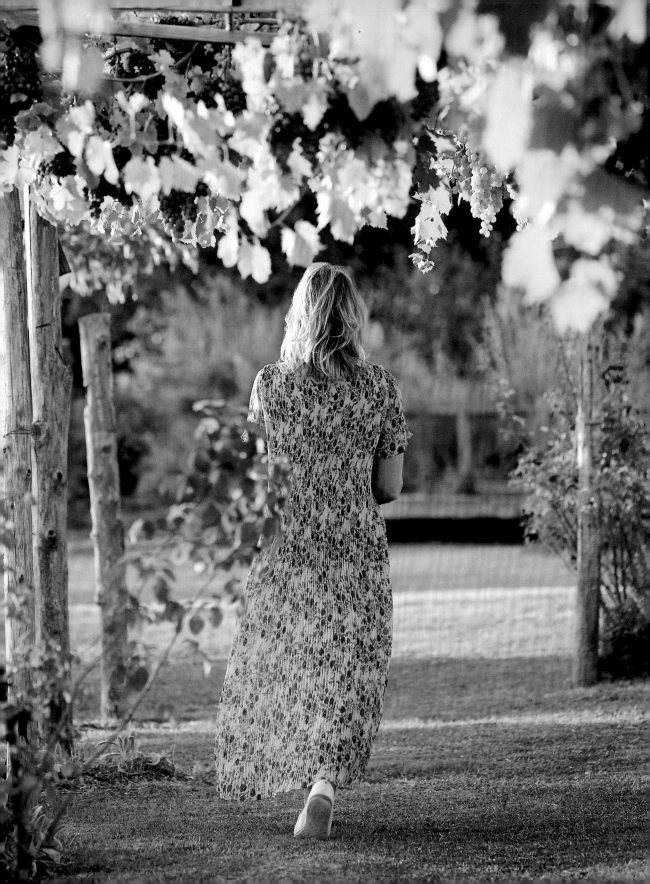

Arrivederci

IN MAY THERE ARE FIREFLIES HERE AT THE VILLA—a theatre
of tiny lights dancing around us on clear evenings. They light up
our lives and show us the way to move more, smile more, touch
more and mingle with others. Life is a celebration.
Unleash the sweet joy.

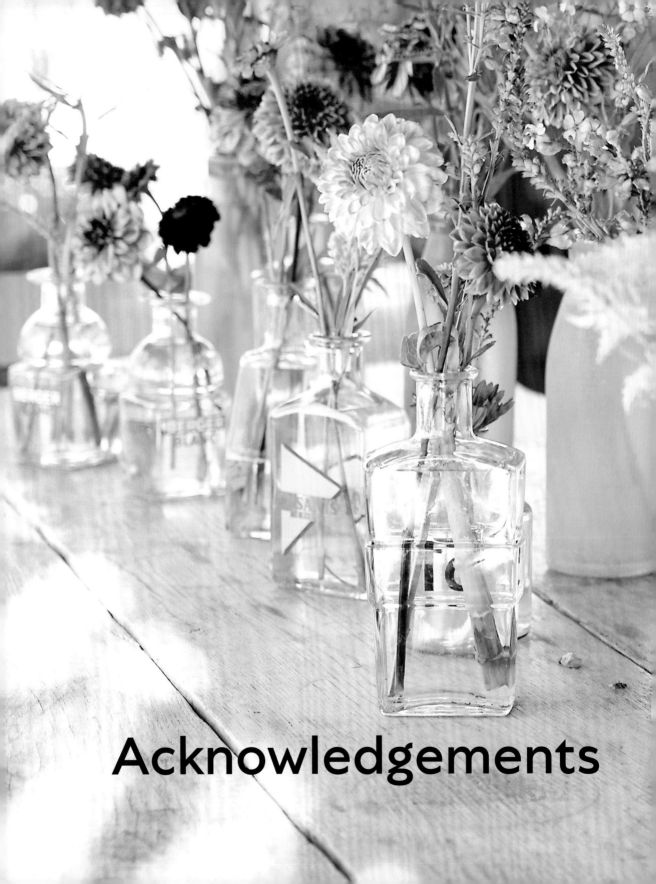

Acknowledgements

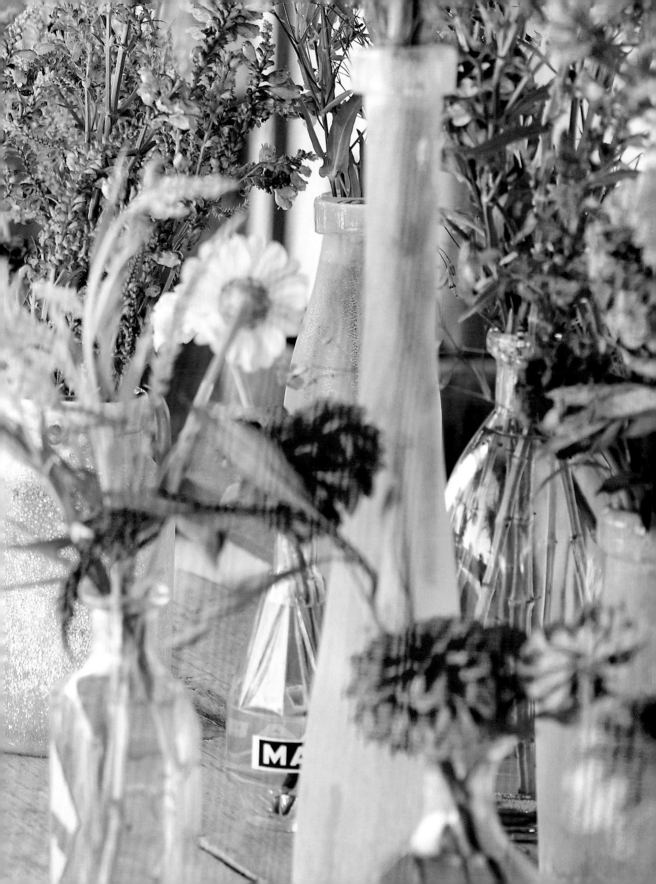

I'd like to thank everyone who came together, like a colourful table of flowers, to create *JOY*. I'm so lucky to be surrounded by such talented souls and I thank you all from the bottom of my heart.

I must begin with my dear husband, Hans. His patience and kindness is boundless. Not a word leaves my writing hut without me first reading it to him. His approval is everything to me.

Big love and gratitude to Jacky Brown. We've been best friends since our late teens, and we do what friends do: support, humour and prop each other up. Together we have run the Tuscan retreats here at the villa and witnessed the emotional and physical changes in our guests during their time with us. As a nutritional therapist, Jacky is the one who provided the scientific knowledge that reinforces the lessons in this book. We have drunk countless mugs of tea around our kitchen tables in London and Tuscany discussing the benefits of optimum nutrition.

A huge thank you to Stacey Van Berkel, whose photographic brilliance illuminates these pages. She called one day, out of the blue, when I was at my desk writing this book; she was coming to Italy on holiday, she said, and she wondered, since we had worked successfully together in the past, whether I was in need of a photographer while she was in the country. I burst into happy tears. I could not think of anyone better to give a visual life to *JOY*. Stacey spent weeks tirelessly capturing life around the villa.

A grateful shout-out to my son Max Rosenstein for the heartfelt portraits of our Tuscan neighbours and to Jacky's son Luke Brown, who photographed his mum and the feisty Angelina in London. A big thanks, too, to Daniela Cesarei, for the stunning shots of foraging, fermenting and our guests cooking up a storm. And much appreciation to international illustrator Michael Hill for his joyful map of Villa Reniella.

I am forever grateful to the villagers of Montefollonico, who allowed us capture their sparkle here; they are my inspiration for how to live a long, happy life. I am also grateful to the local children who patiently gave up their playtime to take part in our photo shoots.

It is impossible to write about the joys of Italian life without discussing food. Thanks to Chef Francesco Bucaletti for bringing his love of the Tuscan cuisine into my kitchen, alongside his sous chefs Marco and Angela. And we will all miss Thomas, who brought so much light to the retreats with his marvelous cocktails.

Every recipe in this book was tested several times by my dear daughter-in-law, Andy Pace (or as she is known here in Italy, Andiamo). A passionate foodie, she not only made sure all the ingredients in the recipes are easily available, but dished up each one to my willing son Max, who happily gave them the thumbs up.

Luca, Maryana, Mimi, Eve, Lalla, Silvia, Pam and the social marvels, Gaye and Rod, are the heartbeat of life at the villa when our retreats are in full swing. A massive thank you to you all.

Along with Jacky Brown, her husband, Steve, was by my side since the day we began the retreats in 2009. We lived together and laughed together . . . a lot. We lost darling Steve before this book was completed. The personification of joy, Steve touched many lives and his energy still infuses these pages.

I am so grateful to my publishing family. This is my eleventh book with Penguin Random House. Each one is like giving birth to a new child: from excitement at the conception, to the hard physical work of nurturing the development, seeking support and endless advice, and then pure happiness when the offspring is launched into the world! Oodles of gratitude, as always, to my editor and friend Anne Collins, whose wisdom brings my vision to these pages. Her patient handholding and ability to grasp the big picture is legendary. I'd also like to thank the book's food editor, Pamela Murray, and its copy editor, Sue Sumeraj, for meticulously checking every aspect of how we conveyed the recipes. I am forever thankful to designer, Lisa Jager, whose creativity had me squealing with delight; to Daniella Zanchetta, for typesetting with care; and also to the book's managing editor, Deirdre Molina, and production whiz Christie Hanson for turning my words and pictures into these gorgeous pages. Thanks, too, to my publicist Dan French for helping me launch *JOY*.

Warm hugs to all the guests who have stayed at Villa Reniella; special thanks to those who shared their stories with me. You are the inspiration of *JOY*.

And last but not least, my nearest and dearest, my loves, Josh, Max, Fiona, Andy, and, again, my rock, Hans. You are my forever joy.

INDEX

smiling, positive effects of, 308, 311–13

solitude, enjoying, 67, 85, 260

soup, 144, 213; recipe for, 139, 154, 159, 167, 208, 209

stock, 131, 207; in recipe, 139, 159, 167; recipe for, 209

stress, 26, 96, 294; about, 266–69; caffeine and, 224; effects of, 23–24, 216, 284; five-by-five rule for, 278–80; sleep and, 96; solutions for, 106, 190–91, 229, 257, 260, 271, 278, 280–81, 285, 304–5; technology and, 88

T

tai chi, 263

tea, 227–29, 247

technology, 268; addiction to, 288; adverse effects of, 18, 34, 66, 88, 95, 99, 102, 254, 290; healthy relationship with, 294–95; taking a break from, 288, 292, 322

thyme tea, 229

Tomato Pizza, Fresh (recipe), 149–50

tomato sauce, 114, 128, 144; in recipe, 274, 276

tomatoes, 129, 144–46; cooking with, 124, 164; nutritional value of, 146; in recipe, 139, 143, 149–50, 153, 154, 175; sun-dried, 121

touch: comfort-levels with, 300; enjoyment of, 298; healing power of, 302–4; importance of, 305, 323

Travis, Debbie. *See also* Villa Reniella: childhood in Northern England, 135, 161, 177, 201, 227, 282, 288, 301–2; *Design Your Next Chapter* by, 34, 45; Hans Rosenstein, husband of, 24, 40, 64, 66, 76, 88, 128, 220, 235, 250, 323; as model, 76, 91, 125, 250; mother of, 67; son(s) of, 66, 74, 260, 278–79; as TV personality, 104, 250, 278

Trombetti family farm. *See* Villa Reniella

Tuscan cuisine, 28, 114–15, 116, 121, 128, 164. *See also* recipes

Tuscan Gazpacho (recipe), 154

U

Urquhart, Sarah, 290

V

Vegetable Stock (recipe), 209

vegetables, 129–31, 217. *See also* recipes

Villa Reniella: camaraderie at, 34; chef at (*see* Francesco, Chef); classes and workshops at, 162, 165, 178, 193, 242, 263, 271; community of, 55; exercise at, 250; lavender grown at, 106; location of, 114; massages at, 14, 304; meals at, 33–34, 117, 161 (*See also* recipes); meditation at, 262; olive grove at, 178, 250; olive oil produced at, 23, 177; original owners of, 55–56; positive change in guests at, 46, 57, 64, 75, 81, 262–63, 269, 308; recapturing vitality at, 23, 268–69; renovating, 27–28, 46, 79, 92, 250; sharing with guests, 28, 33; suites at, 104

vitality. *See also* elderly people: boosting, 21, 28, 33, 38; concept of, 33; loss of, 23–24, 32, 33, 46; path to, 17; renewed, 311; sleep and, 88; tracking feelings of, 50–51

volunteering, joys of, 65–66

Von Schweinichen, Bolko, 212

W

walking, 253–54, 321

water: flavoured, 231, 235, 319; importance of, 231, 247

weight, body: alcohol's effect on, 232; fatigue and, 97; losing, 89, 213; maintaining healthy, 24, 56, 110, 116, 119, 161, 224, 257, 319; obesity and, 40; portion size and, 125

wine: enjoying meals with, 128, 153, 203, 220; fermentation of, 193; flavouring meat with, 203; moderate enjoyment of, 24, 34, 77, 109, 220, 232, 235; preventing overindulgence in, 292, 318–19; pros and cons of, 232; qualities of, 182; in recipe, 171, 175, 241; sharing together, 33, 40, 59, 65, 81, 85, 117, 144, 280; unhealthy habits around, 23, 88, 109, 229, 266; Vin Santo, 57

Y

yoga, 23, 64, 263, 285, 316, 321; benefits of, 109, 111, 257, 284; at Villa Reniella, 8, 253, 260

Z

zucchini, 129, 135, 154; in recipe, 139, 154, 167, 195

zuppa di ceci. See Chickpea Soup (recipe)

DEBBIE TRAVIS is an international television icon, a bestselling author, a newspaper columnist, a sought-after public speaker and the centre of a small business empire. Her shows, *Debbie Travis' Painted House*, *Debbie Travis' Facelift*, *From The Ground Up* and *All For One*—and most recently the six-part documentary, *La Dolce Debbie*, have been seen in Canada, the United States and 80 other countries. She has authored ten previous books (eight on decorating); Oprah has called her "the master of paint and plaster." Having stepped back from TV producing, she gets to relax, just a little, running a luxury boutique hotel where like-minded women can experience the Tuscan lifestyle at her Girls' Getaways and a 100-acre farm where she produces an organic extra virgin olive oil and a variety of lavender products. Debbie shares her journey with her husband, Hans, and two sons, Josh and Max.

JACKY BROWN is a graduate of the London College of Naturopathic Medicine, a qualified Nutritional Therapist, Dip CNM, registered with BANT (British Association of Nutritional Therapists), CNHC and the ANP. Jacky lives with her family in England.

STACEY VAN BERKEL is a passionate creator of beautiful images who has travelled all over the world in search of them. Her work has been featured in numerous international magazines and ad campaigns. She lives in North Carolina.

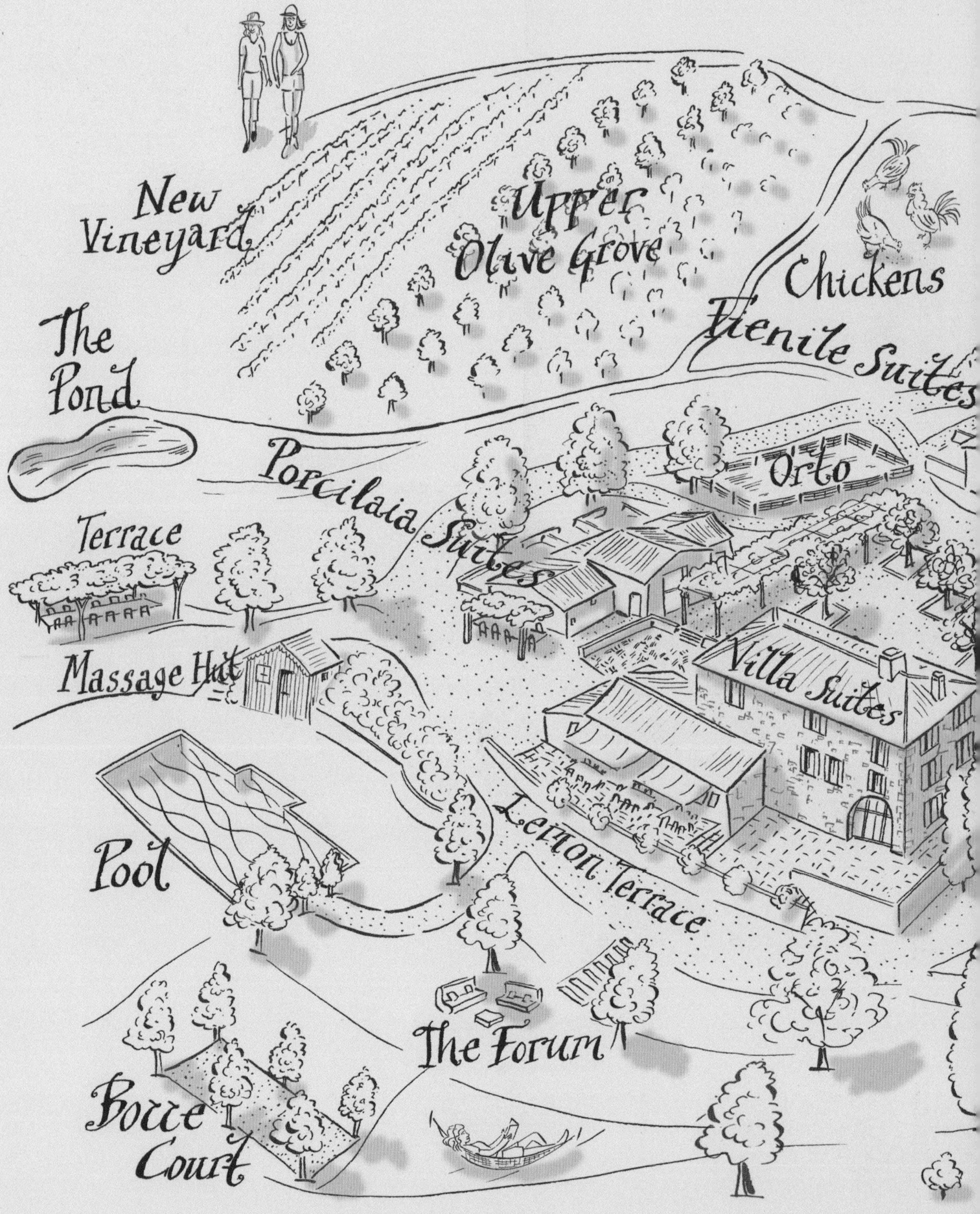
New Vineyard
Upper Olive Grove
Chickens
The Pond
Fienile Suites
Porcilaia Suites
Orto
Terrace
Massage Hut
Villa Suites
Pool
Lemon Terrace
The Forum
Bocce Court